NEW ACTIVITIES IN THE DOPAMINE AGONIST FIELD

NEW ACTIVITIES IN THE DOPAMINE AGONIST FIELD

The Proceedings of a Special Symposium held at the First Congress of the International Society of Gynecological Endocrinology, Crans Montana, Switzerland, March 1988

Edited by
G. M. Besser
St Bartholomew's Hospital, London

The Parthenon Publishing Group
International Publishers in Science & Technology

Casterton Hall, Carnforth,
Lancs, LA6 2LA, U.K.

120 Mill Road, Park Ridge,
New Jersey, U.S.A.

Published in the UK and Europe by
The Parthenon Publishing Group Ltd.
Casterton Hall
Carnforth, Lancs. LA6 2LA   ISBN: 1-85070-197-0

Published in North America by
The Parthenon Publishing Group Inc.
120 Mill Road
Park Ridge
New Jersey, NJ, USA   ISBN: 0-940813-44-0

Copyright © 1988 The Parthenon Publishing Group Ltd.

No part of this publication may be reproduced, stored in a retrieval system, or transmitted in any form or by any means, electronic, mechanical, photocopying, recording or otherwise, without prior permission from the publishers.

Typeset by Lasertext Ltd., Stretford, Manchester
Printed and bound in Great Britain by
Butler & Tanner Ltd, Frome and London

Contents

	List of principal contributors	9
1.	Introduction G. M. Besser	11
2.	CV 205-502, a novel octahydrobenzo[g]quinoline with potent, specific and long-lasting dopamine agonist properties R.C. Gaillard, J. Brownell, K. Abeywickrama and A.F. Muller	13
3.	CV 205-502, a new long-acting dopamine agonist for the treatment of hyperprolactinemia: clinical experience and hormonal findings in a 3-month study in hyperprolactinemic women P.F.M. van der Heijden, R. Rolland, R.E. Lappøhn, R.S. Corbeij, W.B.K.M.V. de Goeij and J. Brownell	27
4.	Oral and parenteral dopamine agonists: comparative effects K. von Werder, J. Schopohl and G. Mehltretter	35
5.	The use of two injectable long-acting bromocriptine preparations (Parlodel® LA and Parlodel® LAR, Sandoz) in patients with prolactinoma F. Cavagnini, C. Maraschini, M. Moro, M. de Martin, C. Invitti, A. Brunani and I. Lancranjan	47
6.	Parlodel® SRO®: an oral modified release formulation of bromocriptine with improved tolerability J. Drewe, E. Abisch and R. Neeter	59

7. Parlodel® SRO® and prolactinomas: clinical and
   therapeutic aspects
   *D. Ayalon, Y. Wachsman, A. Eshel, N. Eckstein,
   I. Vagman and I. Lancranjan*   71

8. Conclusions
   G. M. Besser   81

   Abstracts   83

   Index   91

List of principal contributors

D. Ayalon
Timsit Institute of Reproductive
  Endocrinology,
Ichilov Hospital,
Tel Aviv,
Israel

G.M. Besser
The Medical College of St
  Bartholomew's Hospital,
West Smithfield,
London,
England

F. Cavagnini
Department of Metabolic Diseases,
University of Sassari,
Italy

J. Drewe
Pharma Development,
Sandoz Ltd,
CH-4002 Basle,
Switzerland

R.C. Gaillard
Department of Medicine,
University Hospital,
CH-1211 Geneva 4,
Switzerland

P.F.M. van der Heijden
Department of Obstetrics and
  Gynecology,
St Radboud University Hospital,
Nijmegen,
The Netherlands

K. von Werder
Department of Medicine Innenstadt,
University of Munich,
8000 München 2,
West Germany

1

Introduction

G. M. Besser

There have been dramatic changes in the understanding of pituitary–hypothalamic function in the 17 years since the first publication describing the lowering of prolactin by the drug bromocriptine. Indeed, then it was not clear that bromocriptine was a dopamine agonist, nor that dopamine could lower prolactin by a direct action on the pituitary without affecting gonadotropins directly. Not only has the appearance of this group of drugs produced great clinical benefit for all patients with reproductive disorders, but there have been great advances in understanding of reproductive physiology as a result. Great benefit has also accrued in acromegaly and in parkinsonism.

Many alternative drugs have been developed subsequently with similar actions in an attempt to provide improved bioavailability, lower costs, more specific or wider actions, fewer side-effects or sustained activity. Most have been related ergot compounds. None has yet significantly replaced the original compound, usually because of unacceptable side-effects or toxicity. Most recently new families of substances with specific dopamine agonist qualities but a radically different structure have been investigated. It is the aim of this symposium to survey these new activities and developments.

2

CV 205-502, a novel octahydrobenzo[g]quinoline with potent, specific and long-lasting dopamine agonist properties

R. C. Gaillard, J. Brownell, K. Abeywickrama and A. F. Muller

INTRODUCTION

Ergot alkaloids and their synthetic derivatives have been used in the treatment of a variety of pathophysiological disturbances such as hyperprolactinemic states, acromegaly and Parkinson's disease[1]. Adverse reactions are, however, often a problem at the beginning of the treatment and sometimes persist during chronic therapy. Moreover, the drugs have to be taken several times daily to maintain the therapeutic effect. Hence there is a need for new dopamine agonists with specific and long-lasting action and with a more favorable adverse reaction profile. Efforts have been concentrated on the synthesis of new derivatives and partial structures with the aim of dissecting out the specifically dopaminomimetic pharmacophore. Accordingly, CV 205-502, a structure which superimposes the linear benzo[g]quinoline segment of apomorphine on the substituted pyrrolo[3,4-g]quinoline moiety of the ergolines has recently been designed[2]. The substance is thus a dopaminomimetic substance which does not possess an ergot structure (Figure 1). The dopaminergic properties of CV 205-502 have been demonstrated in vitro and in vivo in animal models[3]. Receptor binding studies have shown that CV 205-502 is a strong D_2 and a

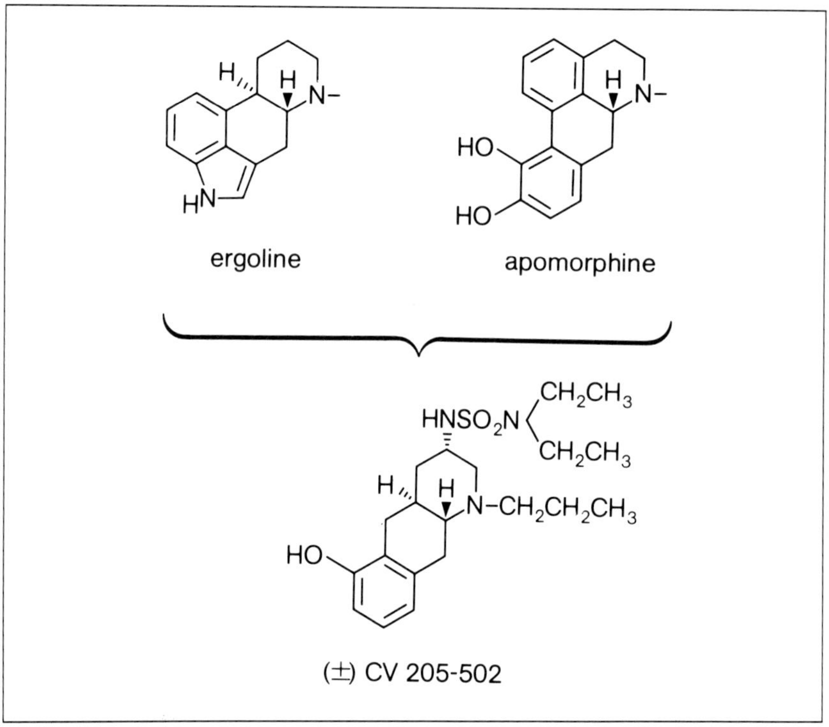

Figure 1 Design of (±) CV 205-502

weak D_1 receptor agonist. In this chapter we have summarized the studies we performed with CV 205-502 in normal young volunteers.

DOSE-RANGING STUDY

The purpose of this study was to assess the effect of single oral doses of CV 205-502 with a view to finding the dose which offers maximal prolactin (PRL) inhibition and optimal tolerance[4].

A group of ten healthy male volunteers participated in this study. They received placebo treatment followed by succeeding higher doses of CV 205-502. Single oral doses of 0.01, 0.02, 0.03, 0.04, 0.06 and 0.08 mg were given to eight subjects per dose and seven subjects received 0.09 mg. The subjects remained the same for the doses 0.01–0.06 mg. An interval of 1 week separated each treatment. Blood sampling for analysis of prolactin (PRL) was performed before and 1, 2, 4, 6, 8 and 24 hours following capsule ingestion.

Mean area under curves (AUCs) for PRL for each dose group are represented in Table 1. Plasma PRL concentrations were lowered dose-dependently, compared with the placebo control (Figures 2, 3).

Table 1 Effect of CV 205-502 on plasma prolactin over a period of 8 hours compared to placebo effect. Mean (± SEM) AUCs for plasma prolactin concentrations (0–8 h) for each drug dose group

Dose of CV 205-502 (mg)	Mean AUCs (0–8 h) for PRL (ng/ml)	
	Placebo	CV 205-502
0.01	41.9 ± 4.6	31.2 ± 2.3
0.02	41.9 ± 4.6	27.4 ± 1.8
0.03	41.9 ± 4.6	25.4 ± 1.8
0.04	41.9 ± 4.6	21.3 ± 2.0
0.06	41.9 ± 4.6	20.5 ± 2.0
0.08	42.6 ± 4.5	23.6 ± 1.5
0.09	41.0 ± 4.3	27.2 ± 0.9

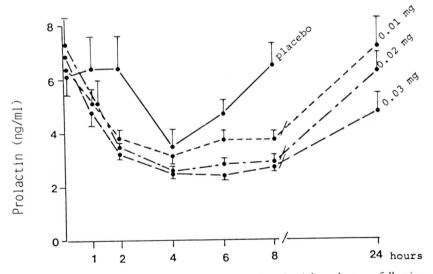

Figure 2 Mean (±SEM) plasma PRL concentrations in eight volunteers following single dose of CV 205-502 (0.01, 0.02 and 0.03 mg) or placebo

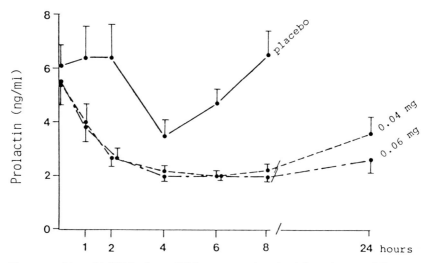

Figure 3 Mean (±SEM) plasma PRL concentrations in eight volunteers following single dose of CV 205-502 (0.04 and 0.06 mg) or placebo

While the 0.04 mg dose produced clinically relevant PRL suppression throughout 8 hours (i.e. PRL values − 60% of placebo), the first indication for a long duration of action was seen following 0.06 mg dose. At this dose, PRL levels were still inhibited 24 hours after capsule ingestion, the values being suppressed by 58% of pretreatment levels. This observation was confirmed by increasing the dose to 0.08 mg and to 0.09 mg (curves not shown).

Side-effects were predominantly mild to moderate headache as well as nausea. One subject only had an episode of vomiting.

This study shows that CV 205-502 is a strong, well tolerated and probably long-acting PRL inhibitor compound[4].

DURATION OF ACTION

Subsequently, we studied the duration of action of CV 205-502 on plasma PRL levels and assessed its effects upon the profile of PRL and growth hormone (GH) elicited during sleep. For this purpose, a single oral dose of 0.06 mg CV 205-502 was given to six healthy volunteers in a double-blind cross-over study with placebo. After capsule ingestion, blood was sampled over 48 hours, including during sleep (from 11 p.m. to 7 a.m.). After 2 hours mean PRL concentrations were markedly inhibited to 66% of their placebo control (Figure 4). Values continued to decline and remained markedly decreased throughout the first 24 hours, abolishing the normal sleep surges of PRL seen after placebo treatment. By 36 hours, PRL values were still suppressed to 47% of their control value, returning to normal levels after 48 hours. These data confirm that CV 205-502 is not only a strong but also a long-acting PRL inhibitor compound, since its effect lasts for at least 24 hours and flattens the sleep PRL profile.

Plasma GH concentrations were slightly and transiently elevated during the first 2–8 hours after capsule ingestion. The sleep pattern, however, had reverted to normal, since slight to strong surges were recorded at midnight and at 2 a.m. corresponding with those following placebo treatment (Figure 5). The transient GH elevations observed at the beginning of the treatment are typical acute effects of dopamine agonist compound[5,6]. The mechanisms of this effect *in vivo* are,

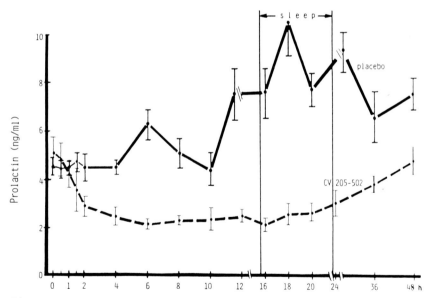

Figure 4 Mean (±SEM) plasma PRL concentrations in six volunteers during a 48-hour period, including sleep, following a single dose of 0.06 mg CV 205-502 or placebo

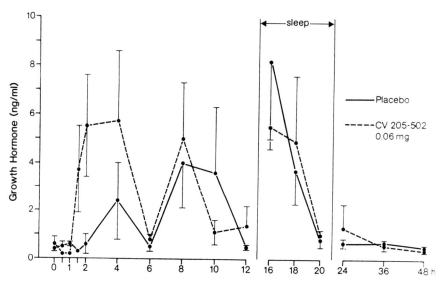

Figure 5 Mean (±SEM) plasma GH concentrations in six volunteers during a 48-hour period, including during sleep, following a single dose of 0.06 mg CV 205-502 or placebo

however, not known. They may involve a direct stimulation of somatotropic dopamine receptors, a dopaminergic stimulation of endogenous GRF[7], or a dopamine inhibition of somatostatin neurons.

ENDOCRINE PROFILE OF CV 205-502

This endocrine profile was performed in six of the volunteers receiving the dose of 0.06 mg CV 205-502. Beside the strong PRL inhibition, CV 205-502 inhibited significantly ($p = 0.028$) TSH levels and produced, in four subjects, a slight to moderate, transient GH stimulation similar to that discussed before (Figure 6). No effect, however, was seen on plasma levels of LH, FSH and cortisol, their values remaining comparable with placebo control values.

In order to investigate the site of action of CV 205-502, and to assess its effects on basal *and* stimulated anterior pituitary hormones, while under steady-state influence of CV 205-502, we studied the effect of this compound during a combined anterior pituitary stimulation test performed after 6 days of CV 205-502 administration[8].

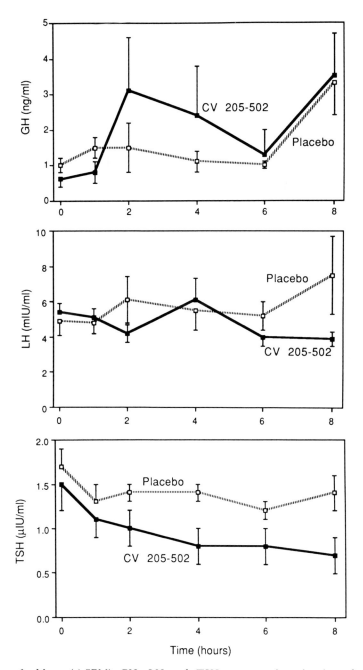

Figure 6 Mean (±SEM) GH, LH and TSH concentrations in six volunteers following a single dose of 0.06 mg CV 205-502 or placebo. Significant inhibition of TSH by CV 205-502 ($p = 0.028$)

Three groups of five men (mean age: 25 years) were treated once daily with CV 205-502 at a dose of 0.04, 0.06 or 0.08 mg/day (doses which suppress PRL by 60–68% over 24 hours). On day 6 of this treatment, a combined anterior pituitary function test was performed using the sequential intravenous administration of the four hypothalamic releasing hormones (100 μg GRF, 100 μg LHRH, 100 μg CRF and 200 μg TRH). 1 month later, the combined anterior pituitary function test was repeated to obtain control values. Blood was sampled before and at regular intervals during 3 hours after the challenge tests for measurement by radioimmunoassay of plasma LH, FSH, testosterone, ACTH, cortisol, TSH, GH and PRL.

All volunteers responded normally to the combined anterior pituitary function test with strong stimulation of all hormones, both under CV 205-502 treatment and after the 1-month washout, with the exception of the PRL response which was largely attenuated during treatment with CV 205-502. Basal PRL levels were significantly reduced 24 hours after the previous CV 205-502 administration (60–80% inhibition), and the magnitude of the PRL response to TRH was significantly decreased in all subjects while under CV 205-502 treatment ($p < 0.05$ and $p < 0.01$). The dopaminergic properties of all three doses were strong enough to block the TRH stimulation (Figure 7). The lactotroph cells appeared to be the only adenohypophyseal cells whose secretory activity was altered by a direct action of CV 205-502, since the response of all other anterior pituitary cells to their respective hypothalamic releasing hormones remained unaffected by CV treatment. Indeed the responses of the pituitary-adrenal, -thyroid and -gonadal axes were unaffected by CV 205-502. Despite the recently described coexistence of GRF and dopamine in neurons of the tuberoinfundibular system, suggesting a possible interaction between both compounds in the control of GH release[9], CV 205-502 did not consistently influence the GH response to GRF[8]. Although, as discussed before, the precise mechanism by which dopamine controls GH secretion in man remains speculative, it has to be emphasized that the new non-ergot dopamine agonist CV 205-502 has no important action on GH secretion in normal man.

The absence of effect of CV 205-502 on both basal and stimulated gonadotropin and testosterone levels (Figure 8) is important in regard to the potential use of CV 205-502 to treat men and women with

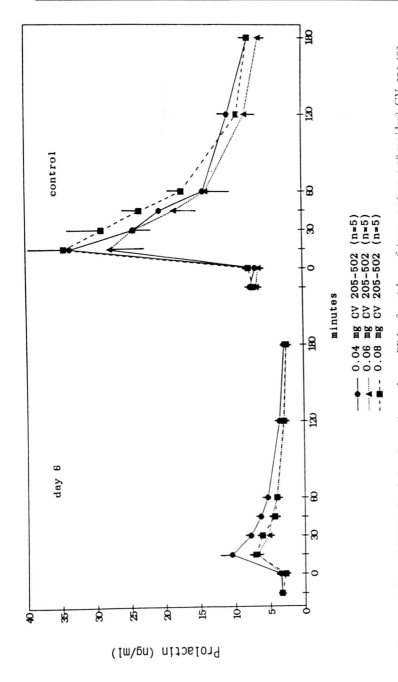

Figure 7 Effect of TRH stimulation (200 μg) on plasma PRL after 6 days of (0.04, 0.06 or 0.08 mg/day) CV 205-502 administration (left) and during the control day (right). (Mean ± SEM)

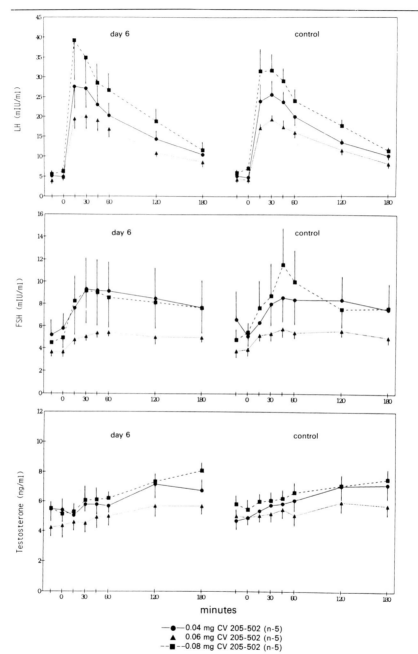

Figure 8 Effect of LHRH stimulation (100 μg) on plasma LH, FSH and testosterone after 6 days of CV 205-502 administration (left) and during the control day (right). (Mean ± SEM)

hyperprolactinemia and impaired sexual function.

Despite the slight inhibitory effect observed after a single dose of CV 205-502 on basal plasma TSH levels (Figure 6), 6 days of CV 205-502 administration did not affect basal and TRH-stimulated TSH levels (Figure 9).

CV 205-502 had no effect on the pituitary-adrenal axis, since both basal and CRF-stimulated ACTH and cortisol levels were not affected by any of the three drug doses.

TOLERANCE

CV 205-502 was well tolerated by the healthy volunteers, since adverse reactions (headache and nausea) were minimal and were reported mainly with the two highest doses. At all dose levels, supine blood pressure and pulse rate measurements remained largely unchanged from placebo control values. Clinically relevant blood pressure decreases were seen only occasionally at the highest dose levels (0.08 and 0.09 mg). Pulse rate remained essentially unchanged from those following placebo, even when blood pressure decreases were recorded. This good tolerance after the single dose study was confirmed by a multiple-dose study in which single doses from 0.02 to 0.1 mg CV 205-502 or placebo were given daily for 5 days to eight healthy volunteers per treatment group. As indicated in Table 2 adverse reactions observed in this study consisted predominantly of nausea and headache. Orthostatic blood pressure decreases were recorded in five subjects at the highest dose levels.

In conclusion our studies demonstrate that CV 205-502 has strong, well tolerated and long-acting dopamine agonist properties and implicates the pituitary as its major site of action. The data suggest also that the lactotropic cells are the only adenohypophyseal cells whose secretory activity is altered by a direct action of this dopaminergic compound. This new dopamine agonist, which does not possess an ergot structure, needs now to be tested in pathological situations. Because of its new design, CV 205-502 may be effective in case of ergot-derivative resistance or intolerance[10-12] and could probably be prescribed at a once-daily dosage.

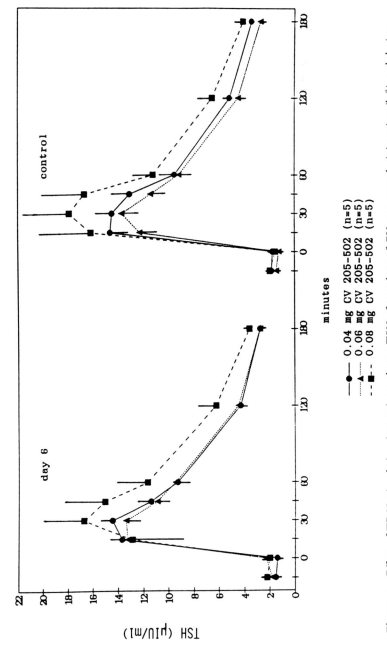

Figure 9 Effect of TRH stimulation (200 μg) on plasma TSH after 6 days of CV 205-502 administration (left) and during the control day (right). (Mean ± SEM)

Table 2 Number of subjects with commonly reported adverse reactions during 6-day observation under CV 205-502 treatment

Adverse reaction [body system]	Treatment					
	0.02 mg (n = 5)	0.04 mg (n = 5)	0.06 mg (n = 5)	0.08 mg (n = 5)	0.1 mg (n = 5)	Placebo (n = 15)
Weakness, faintness	—	1	2	1	2	—
Headache [CNS]	1	—	1	3	3	7
Nausea (vomiting) [Gastrointestinal]	—	—	2(—)	3(1)	5(3)	2(1)

ACKNOWLEDGEMENTS

The authors wish to thank Mrs D. Turnill and C. Chauffat-Rabère for their excellent technical assistance. This work was supported by the Swiss National Science Foundation (grant No 3.814.084) and Sandoz Ltd, Basle, Switzerland. Figures 2, 3, 4 and 5 are reproduced from ref. 4 and Figures 7, 8 and 9 from ref. 8.

REFERENCES

1. Vance, M.L., Evans, W.A. and Thorner, M.O. (1984). Bromocriptine. *Ann. Intern. Med.*, **100**, 78–91
2. Nordmann, R. and Petcher, T.J. (1985). Octahydrobenzo[g]quinolines: potent dopamine agonists which show the relationship between ergolines and apomorphine. *J. Med. Chem.*, **28**, 367–75
3. Gaillard, R.C., Nordmann, R., Petcher, T.J. and Brownell, J. (1986). A novel octahydrobenzo[g]quinoline, CV 205-502, with potent dopamine agonist properties. In Molinatti, G.M. and Martini, L. (eds.) *Endocrinology 1985*. pp 305–8. (Amsterdam: Elsevier Science Publishers)
4. Gaillard, R.C. and Brownell, J. (1988). Hormonal effect of CV 205-502, a novel octahydrobenzo[g]quinoline, with potent and long-acting dopamine agonist properties. *Life Sci.*, (In press)
5. Flückiger, E. (1978). Ergot alkaloids and the modulation of hypothalamic function. In Cox, B., Morris I.D. and Weston, A.H. (eds.) *Pharmacology of the Hypothalamus*. pp 137–60. (London: Macmillan)
6. DiChiara, G. et al. (1978). Stimulation of regulatory dopamine receptors by bromocriptine (CB 154). *Pharmacology*, **16** (suppl.1), 135–42

7. Leebaw, W.F., Lee, L.A. and Woolf, P.D. (1978). Dopamine affects basal and augmented pituitary growth hormone secretion. *J. Clin. Endocrinol. Metab.*, **47**, 480
8. Gaillard, R.C., Abeywickrama, K., Brownell, J. and Muller, A.F. (1988). Specific effect of CV 205-502, a potent non-ergot dopamine agonist, during a combined anterior pituitary function test. *Clin. Endocrinol. Metab.*, (In press)
9. Meister, B., Hökfelt, T., Vale, W., Sawchenko, P.E., Swanson, L. and Goldstein, M. (1986). Coexistence of tyrosine hydroxylase and growth hormone-releasing factor in a subpopulation of tuberoinfundibular neurons of the rat. *Neuroendocrinology*, **42**, 237–47
10. Grossman, A., Bouloux, P.M.G., Loneragan, R., Rees, L.H., Wass, J.A.H. and Besser, G.M. (1985). Comparison of the clinical activity of mesulergine and pergolide in the treatment of hyperprolactinemia. *Clin. Endocrinol. (Oxf.)*, **22**, 611–16
11. Grossman, A. and Besser, G.M. (1985). Prolactinomas. *Br. Med. J.*, **290**, 182–4
12. Ahmet, S.R. and Shaled, S.M. (1986). Discordant responses of prolactinoma to two different dopamine agonists. *Clin. Endocrinol. (Oxf.)*, **24**, 421–6

3

CV 205-502, a new long-acting dopamine agonist for the treatment of hyperprolactinemia: clinical experience and hormonal findings in a 3-month study in hyperprolactinemic women

P.F.M. van der Heijden, R. Rolland, R.E. Lappøhn, R.S. Corbeij, W.B.K.M.V. de Goeij and J. Brownell

---

INTRODUCTION

Hyperprolactinemia is best treated by dopamine agonists such as bromocriptine (Parlodel[R]). Associated with the ergoline structure of these drugs, they may give rise to side-effects and intolerance may be clinically important, although their prolactin lowering effect is excellent[1]. CV 205-502, octahydrobenzo[g]quinoline, (CV) is a new dopamine agonistic drug. The molecular structure (see Figure 1 of Chapter 2) indicates that it is not of the ergot type. Studies in volunteers have shown this drug to exert good prolactin lowering effect accompanied by very few side-effects[2]. Preliminary studies in hyperprolactinemic women have also indicated good prolactin suppressant effects of CV when given once daily at bedtime[3]. The purpose of this study was to ascertain the dosage at which CV exerts a clinically relevant prolactin suppressant effect in hyperprolactinemic women and to assess at regular intervals the safety and tolerance of this compound in hyperprolactinemic women. The study was carried out in two university clinics and two departments of gynecology and obstetrics in large hospitals in The Netherlands.

STUDY DESIGN

41 women suffering from persistent hyperprolactinemia with prolactin persistently above 2000 mU/l agreed to participate in the study. After having received both oral and written information concerning the study, they gave their written informed consent. The study protocol itself had been approved by the different ethical committees of the separate hospitals. In a randomized, prospective and double-blind manner, 20 women received placebo and 21 women CV for the first 4 weeks. The initial starting dose in the active drug-treatment group was 0.05 mg with the possibility of increasing the daily dose if necessary by 0.025 mg at 4 and 8 weeks. Hence, the final dosage of CV which could be reached within 3 months in this group was 0.10 mg. The code was broken after 4 weeks and at this time the placebo group started with 0.05 mg. Therefore the maximal dosage which could be reached within the study period in this group was 0.075 mg. All capsules were taken once daily at bedtime. After having been selected for the study, the women were seen every second week throughout the study period. In a subgroup of 12 of these patients, a pituitary challenge test with TRH was performed before the study and at 4 weeks of treatment (prior to breaking the code) in six women receiving CV and six women receiving placebo. They all were given 200 μg TRH in 2 ml saline and at frequent intervals serum samples were taken for prolactin and TSH measurements. Both hormones were measured by radioimmunoassay. During the study prolactin was measured every second week as were parameters like blood pressure (both standing and supine), pulse rate and weight. Safety parameters including hematology, blood chemistry, urine analysis and ECG determinations were carried out every 4 weeks.

In Table 1 the pretreatment findings are shown in the patients and there were no obvious differences between the two groups. 38 of the 41 women had previously received dopamine agonist therapy with bromocriptine. Several of them showed poor tolerance to this drug and this was the main reason for participation in this study.

Table 1 Pretreatment findings in 41 hyperprolactinemic women with serum prolactin persistently above 2000 mU/l previous to treatment

Item	CV 205-502 starters (n = 21)	Placebo starters (n = 20)
Age (years)	31.6 (±1.54)	32.3 (±1.33)
Height (cm)	167.0 (±1.27)	166.1 (±1.83)
Weight (kg)	64.4 (±1.8)	67.6 (±2.0)
Parity (n)		
multiparae	12	11
nulliparae	9	9
Galactorrhea (n)	12	12
Infertility (> 1 year, n)	10	10
Amenorrhea (>6 month, n)	11	14
Oligomenorrhea (n)	6	5
Previous dopamine agonist therapy (n)	20	18

RESULTS

Figure 1 depicts the prolactin responses to TRH in both subgroups before drug intake and during treatment either with placebo or CV. Prior to treatment both groups showed a blunted or absent response to TRH. During treatment at 4 weeks the placebo group showed the same response, whereas in the six women treated with CV a significant suppression of serum prolactin had occurred prior to TRH administration. In response to TRH a significant increase in serum prolactin occurred with a maximum at 30 min with thereafter a gradual decrease.

Prior to and during treatment the TSH response in the separate groups was identical (not shown).

20 women normalized their serum prolactin (prolactin below 750 mU/l) while being treated with 0.05 mg CV. Ten had normalized their prolactin at a CV dosage of 0.075 mg and three women had normalized their prolactin while taking 0.1 mg CV at the 3-month analysis. Eight women did not normalize their prolactin within this dosage scheme and were treated beyond the period of 3 months. Their prolactin finally normalized on a dosage of CV of 0.125 or 0.150 mg.

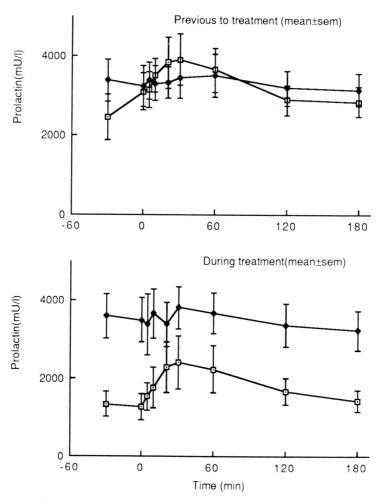

Figure 1 Serum prolactin levels previous to and during a TRH challenge test in six placebo treated women and six CV 205-502 treated women (200 μg at time 0). Prior to treatment (upper panel) and during treatment at 4 weeks (lower panel). Open squares: CV-treated women, closed squares: placebo-treated women

Figure 2 shows the serum prolactin concentrations measured in the two groups throughout the study period. The grouping into those women receiving either 0.05, 0.075 or 0.1 mg at 12 weeks has been

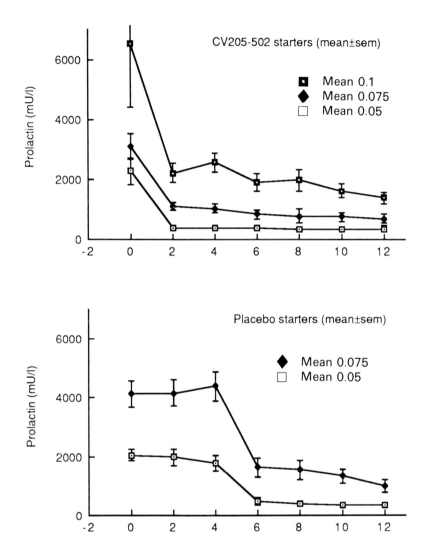

Figure 2 Serum prolactin levels (mean ± SEM) in CV 205-502 treated women (upper panel) and in CV 205-502 treated women who received placebo tablets for the first 4 weeks (lower panel). The groups have been constructed retrospectively by grouping women at 12 weeks who at that time received either 0.05 mg, 0.075 mg or 0.1 mg CV 205-502

performed retrospectively. This figure clearly suggests that the higher the initial prolactin level previous to treatment, the higher the dose of CV needed to return prolactin to normal. The figure also clearly indicates that serum prolactin is not influenced by placebo treatment.

Prior to treatment 25 women suffered from secondary amenorrhea. At the end of the observation period (12 weeks) 19 of these women had shown one or more menstrual episodes. During the first 4 weeks of treatment six women receiving placebo and participating in the challenge test showed persistent anovulation whereas three of the six women in the CV group were in the postovulatory phase of their (re-)initiated cycle at 4 weeks.

24 women suffered from galactorrhea prior to treatment. At the end of the observation period 19 of these women were cured or the galactorrhea had improved substantially. Six women still suffered from galactorrhea and actually in three of these women the galactorrhea had worsened.

Two women conceived during the observation period, one of these pregnancies went to full term with the delivery of a healthy baby; unfortunately the second pregnancy ended in a spontaneous abortion.

Findings concerning side-effects are shown in Table 2. Headache and nausea were present in the CV group at the second week of treatment but tended to disappear as treatment continued. The observed side-effects were slight to moderate in severity and – as shown from the table – short lasting in nature. In no case was discontinuation of the study necessary. Of the 38 women previously treated with

Table 2 Side-effects reported during the first 4 weeks of treatment with CV 205-502 (21 women) or placebo (20 women). (x) indicates the number of women who mentioned the same side-effect at both 2 and 4 weeks

	CV 205-502		Placebo	
	2 weeks	4 weeks	2 weeks	4 weeks
Headache	7	2(1)	4	4(2)
Nausea	6	2(2)	1	1
Dizziness	1	1	1	
Tiredness	1	1(1)		1
Acne			1	

bromocriptine, 28 responded as well to CV as to their previous treatment while ten responded better to CV. These ten had shown poor tolerance to bromocriptine.

As far as the safety parameters are concerned, no drug-attributable abnormalities in any measure of physical, ECG or laboratory blood and urine tests were seen during the 3 months' study, nor did blood pressure and pulse measurements (supine and standing) indicate a significant effect of this drug on these parameters.

CONCLUSIONS

CV 205-502 has been tested in 41 hyperprolactinemic volunteers in a dose-finding study. Within the range tested, the drug showed good prolactin lowering effects although eight of the 41 women needed higher dosages before becoming normoprolactinemic. Since the tolerance and the safety of the drug are excellent, it is suggested that a quickly titrated dose of 0.075 mg or higher could be given. The higher the prolactin level previous to treatment, the higher the dose of CV 205-502 necessary to obtain normoprolactinemia seems to be. It is therefore suggested that in women with high prolactin levels the dosage should be increased rather rapidly.

Parallel to the prolactin lowering effect of the drug, amenorrhea and galactorrhea disappeared as expected. In the women who underwent a TRH challenge test a clear trend towards a strong release of prolactin after TRH while treated with CV 205-502 was obvious. This is in disagreement with findings in normoprolactinemic volunteers treated with the same drug, where this response was blunted[4]. It is, however, in agreement with findings in postpartum women treated with bromocriptine for the purpose of inhibition of lactation. Also in these women a trend towards strong prolactin response is seen when TRH is administered within 3 weeks after delivery and while on bromocriptine[5]. *In vitro* studies by Pasteels[6] also showed that although spontaneous prolactin release is inhibited when dopamine agonists are added to the culture medium, additional TRH gives rise to increased release of prolactin. It is therefore suggested that although dopamine agonists block the release of the hormone at the level of the lactotrophs, these cells remain capable of responding to TRH for at least 3–4 weeks.

It is concluded that the profile of CV 205-502 as judged from the presented studies is not different from other dopamine agonistic drugs like bromocriptine despite the non-ergot structure of the drug. The prolactin lowering capacity seems very promising and it is suggested that an early treatment dose should be at least 0.075 mg. Further dose finding studies must determine the exact starting dose. Since the patients showed good tolerance to the drug and once daily administration at bedtime was sufficient to maintain adequate prolactin suppression over a 24-hour period, it is suggested that this compound may become a welcome alternative to dopamine agonistic drugs of the ergot type. This is specially indicated by the fact that ten of the 41 women who in the past showed poor tolerance to bromocriptine could continue the intake of CV 205-502 with few or absent side-effects.

REFERENCES

1. Thorner, M.O., Flückiger, E. and Calne, D.B. (eds.) (1980) *Bromocriptine. A Clinical and Pharmacological Review.* (New York: Raven Press)
2. Gaillard, R., Nordmann, R., Petcher, T.J. and Brownell, J. (1986). A novel octahydrobenzo[g]quinoline, CV 205-502, with potent dopamine agonist properties. In Molinatti, G.M. and Martini, L. (eds.) *Endocrinology 1985.* pp. 305–8. (Amsterdam: Elsevier Science)
3. Bergh, T., Rasmussen, C., Wide, L. and Brownell, J. (1988). CV 205-502: A new long-acting drug for inhibition of prolactin hypersecretion. *Clin. Endocrinol.,* (In press)
4. Gaillard, R.C., Brownell, J. and Abeywickrama, K. (1986). Specific effect of CV 205-502, a potent dopamine agonist, on prolactin secretion combined pituitary function test with TRH, CRH, GRH and LHRH. *1st International Congress of Neuroendocrinology,* San Francisco, CA. July 1986. Abstract no. 138, p. 57
5. Vemer, H.M. and Rolland, R. (1981). The dynamics of prolactin secretion during the puerperium in women. *Clin. Endocrinol.,* **15**, 155–63
6. Pasteels, J.L., Danguy, A., Frérotte, M. and Ectors, F. (1971). Inhibition de la sécrétion de prolactine par l'ergocornine et la 2-Br-alpha-ergocryptine: action directe sur l'hypophyse en culture. *Ann. Endocrinol. (Paris),* **32**, 188–92

4
Oral and parenteral dopamine agonists: comparative effects

K. von Werder, J. Schopohl and G. Mehltretter

INTRODUCTION

Ergot alkaloids and their derivatives have been used extensively in the past and have become treatment of choice for patients with hyperprolactinemia[1]. The prolactin inhibitory effect of ergot derivatives is mediated by the dopamine-2-receptors at the pituitary level, though these drugs interact also with adrenoreceptors and serotonin-receptors[2,3].

Ergot alkaloids with dopaminergic activity can be divided into three groups according to the structure (Figure 1). Bromocriptine belongs to the lysergic acid amines and contains a tripeptide[2,3]. The most important prolactin inhibitors of the clavines family are metergoline, pergolide and lergotrile. The use of the latter has been abandoned because of side-effects. The most important dopaminergic compounds of the 8α-aminoergolines are lisuride, the transdihydroderivative terguride[4] and cabergoline[5].

The various dopamine agonists differ in duration of action and prolactin lowering potency. Pergolide, which has been used already in clinical trials, is more potent and has also a longer duration of action after oral administration compared to lisuride, bromocriptine and mesulergine[6]. Recently even longer acting drugs like cabergoline have been introduced into the treatment of hyperprolactinemia as investigative drugs[5,7].

Table 1 shows the approximate equivalent dosages of the various dopamine (DA) agonists in respect to their prolactin lowering efficacy,

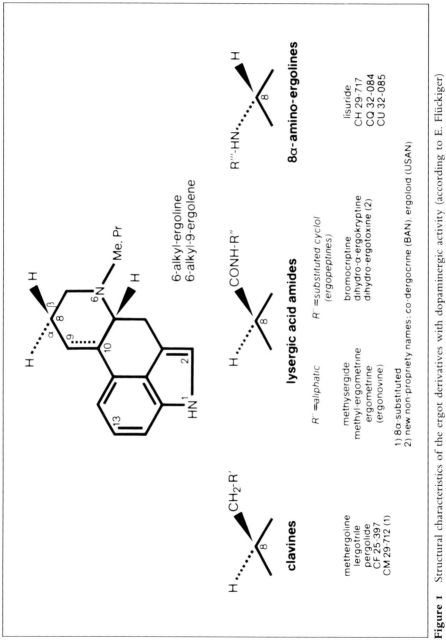

Figure 1 Structural characteristics of the ergot derivatives with dopaminergic activity (according to E. Flückiger)

Table 1 Approximate equivalent dosages of dopamine agonists (PRL-lowering effect)

Bromocriptine	1.0
Dihydroergocriptine	2.0
Mesulergine	0.2
Cabergoline	0.1
Terguride	0.1
Lisuride	0.08
Pergolide	0.01

when compared with bromocriptine on a weight basis. Though there are drugs, which are more than 100 times more potent than bromocriptine, the higher potency has no obvious advantages, because it also means that these drugs have a higher potency in respect to side-effects. Thus, it has never been clearly demonstrated in controlled studies that one dopamine agonist has less side-effects in comparable prolactin lowering dosages compared to another, be it more or less potent[5]. However, it has been repeatedly suggested that in individual patients switching from one dopamine agonist to another may lead to better tolerance[8]. The case reports, however, are difficult to evaluate because of the significant spontaneous fluctuation of basal prolactin (PRL) levels[1].

ORAL ADMINISTRATION OF DOPAMINE AGONISTS

Most of our knowledge in medical treatment of hyperprolactinemia has derived from the experience with oral administration of bromocriptine, which has been specifically developed as a prolactin inhibitor[3], soon after establishment of human prolactin as a separate anterior pituitary hormone[2]. Though oral bromocriptine is very effective in patients with hyperprolactinemia[9] or prolactinomas[10] and should serve as the 'gold standard' when other dopamine agonists are evaluated in comparison[6], there are occasionally patients who may not tolerate bromocriptine because of side-effects. These adverse effects are intrinsic to DA-receptor stimulation and include hypotension and gastrointestinal disturbances, headaches and nasal stuffiness, which are seldom severe and mostly transitory. Cold-sensitive digital vasospasm has been observed in up to 30% of acromegalic patients[3]. Though these symptoms are never severe and disappear if the drug is withdrawn, they can make treatment of prolactinomas or hyperprolactinemic sterility occasionally impossible.

We have initially used CU 32-085, mesulergine, which has been withdrawn from clinical investigation because of side-effects observed in animals, as an alternative for bromocriptine in patients, who did not tolerate the latter[8].

Table 2 shows that this drug may be effective in long-term treatment in patients with macroadenomas in whom stable reduction of PRL levels could not be achieved with bromocriptine.

Lisuride, the second drug, which appeared on the market in most countries, has no obvious advantages compared to bromocriptine[11,12]. Thus, when the efficacy of long-term treatment with lisuride in a group of macroprolactinoma patients was compared with bromocriptine treatment no significant difference was found (Figure 2). However, individual patients were observed, who did not tolerate lisuride but bromocriptine and vice versa in prolactin normalizing dosages[1].

The transdihydroderivative terguride, which is less effective than lisuride, was shown to be tolerated better in individual patients who did not tolerate either bromocriptine or lisuride in prolactin normalizing dosages[4,13]. However, there are no controlled double-blind studies and a placebo effect cannot be excluded. This phenomenon, that individual dopamine agonists, among them the recently introduced very potent compounds, may show a dissociation of prolactin suppressing effect and the intrinsic side-effects of dopamine agonists in individual patients, has been demonstrated by several authors[1,8,13]. However, there is no way to predict if this or that compound may be better tolerated in DA-agonist-sensitive patients unless they are tried out. Though those patients may benefit from switching to another drug, patients in whom the prolactinoma is insensitive to dopamine agonists have no benefit if another dopamine agonist is used, the dosage is raised, or a parenteral route of drug administration is chosen[14]. Thus, a high dosage of oral bromocriptine and an extremely high parenteral Parlodel® LA-dosage had no further effect on PRL levels in a patient with a malignant prolactinoma and spinal and cerebellar metastases (Figure 3).

Table 2 Long-term therapy with bromocriptine (BC) and mesulergine (CU 32-085). Human prolactin (hPRL) levels in ten patients with hyperprolactinemia before and during bromocriptine therapy and during therapy with CU 32-085 (von Werder et al.[8])

Patient	Sex and age	hPRL before therapy (μU/ml)	hPRL BC-therapy (μU/ml)	BC-dosage (mg/day)	hPRL CU 32-085 (μU/ml)	CU 32-085 dosage (mg/day)
S.F.	f 29	3 370	not tolerated	—	175	0.5
F.H.	f 28	5 465	1 980	3.75	443	2.5
S.S.	f 31	436 000	not tolerated	—	9 212	1.5
R.K.	f 30	4 518	230	90.0	100	3.0
D.K.	f 31	20 000	2 637	60.0	1 428	3.0
H.K.	f 32	2 700	578	5.0	35	1.0
P.R.	m 35	41 000	876	10.0	114	1.5
A.K.	m 61	297 255	4 000	30.0	284	3.0
N.S.	m 60	30 289	237	10.0	92	0.5
H.R.	m 35	375 000	183 450	30.0	23 000	4.5

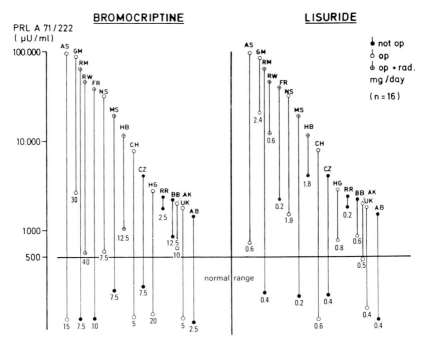

Figure 2 Effect of long-term bromocriptine and lisuride administration on hPRL levels in the same 16 patients. The minimal duration of treatment with a final maximal dose (mg per day at the foot of each bar) was 2 months

PARENTERAL DOPAMINE AGONIST ADMINISTRATION

Recently two injectable forms of bromocriptine, Parlodel® LA (long acting) and Parlodel® LAR (long acting repeatable), have been developed for intramuscular injection (Sandoz Ltd.)[15]. Marked reduction of PRL secretion is seen 3 hours after injection. Furthermore, persisting suppression of PRL secretion was found for about 6 weeks after a single intramuscular injection of 50 mg Parlodel LA[15]. This was accompanied by similar adverse effects as seen after oral administration of bromocriptine. Though dopamine agonistic intrinsic side-effects were seen on the day after injection, adverse effects lasting over a whole week were a rare event[15-17]. After development of Parlodel LAR chronic treatment of patients with macro- and microprolactinomas has been started demonstrating a high normalization rate in both groups

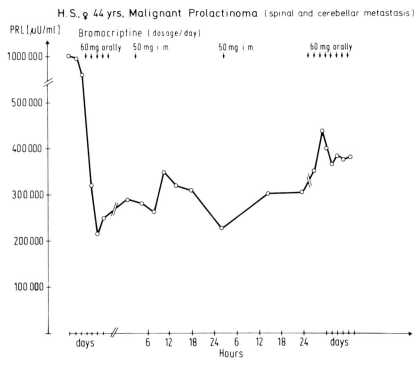

Figure 3 Prolactin levels in a patient with a malignant prolactinoma and a spinal and cerebellar metastasis. Despite a high dosage of parenteral bromocriptine (2 times 50 mg per day) no further lowering of the PRL level could be achieved. This patient finally died because of central complications of the tumor, which was insensitive to bromocriptine (up to 140 mg per day), somatostatin, and cytotoxic therapy[14]

of patients with minor side-effects. As observed after oral bromocriptine treatment[18], rapid tumor shrinkage was also seen after one single intramuscular injection of 50 mg bromocriptine[16]. We have used Parlodel LAR in four patients, in whom we were unable to normalize PRL levels with different oral dopamine agonists, because none of them was tolerated in a dosage to achieve sustained prolactin suppression (Figure 4). The parenteral administration of 50 mg, respectively 100 mg Parlodel LAR caused severe hypotension in two of the patients, which disappeared after 24 hours. In the other two patients no significant adverse effects were recorded, though these patients suffered from severe side-effects

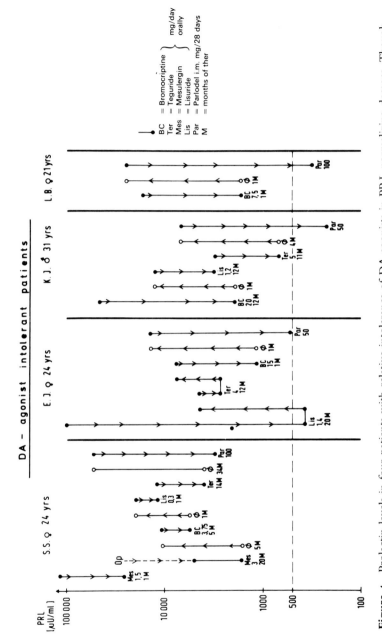

Figure 4 Prolactin levels in four patients with relative intolerance of DA agonists in PRL normalizing dosages. Though the different DA agonists were increased up to the limit of tolerance, PRL levels could not be normalized chronically. Two of these patients had no side-effects after intramuscular injection of Parlodel LAR 50 mg (see Figure 5)

Oral and parenteral dopamine agonists

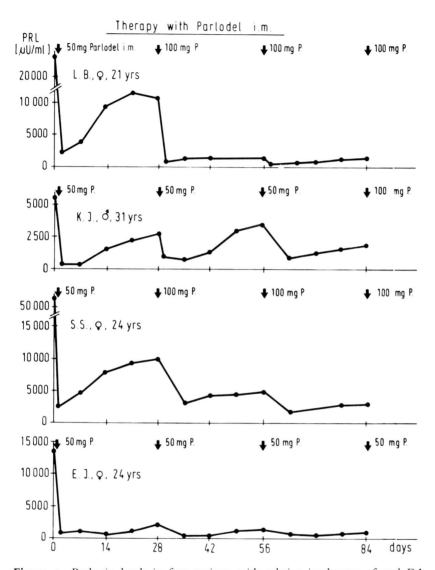

Figure 5 Prolactin levels in four patients with relative intolerance of oral DA agonists after intramuscular injection of 50 and 100 mg Parlodel LAR. Only two patients had adverse effects after the first injection, which diminished and disappeared respectively after the second 100 mg injection. Two patients (S.S., J.E.), who had significant adverse effects after oral DA agonists, had no side-effects at all

when they were taking different DA agonists orally. After administration of Parlodel LAR intramuscularly prolactin levels decreased rapidly and remained lower over 28 days than before treatment (Figure 5). It was of interest that the second intramuscular injection of 100 mg Parlodel LAR did not lead to the same degree of hypotension as the first dosage of 50 mg and had no side-effects in the two others, though all four patients were unable to tolerate oral DA agonists. The PRL levels 24 hours after the second Parlodel LAR injection was significantly lowered compared to the PRL level 24 hours after the first injection. This observation of better tolerance but greater efficacy seems to make this form of dopamine agonist administration very promising.

CONCLUDING REMARKS

Dopamine agonists are the treatment of choice in patients with hyperprolactinemia and prolactinomas. Oral administration of bromocriptine is the most frequently used form of treatment, though some patients may be intolerant of the drug. In these instances alternative dopamine agonists taken orally may be used, since there is an individual but no general dissociation between adverse side-effects and the PRL lowering effect. Since many of these patients do not tolerate any of the oral compounds, which are available for therapy or clinical investigation, parenteral administration of bromocriptine may be indicated, since the latter has been shown to be effective and well tolerated, even in those patients who were unable to take dopamine agonists orally. The parenteral route may also solve problems of compliance which is particularly important in patients with invasive macroprolactinomas expanding into the suprasellar space, where they threaten vision and disturb vital functions.

REFERENCES

1. von Werder, K. (1985). Recent advances in the diagnosis and treatment of hyperprolactinemia. In Imura, H. (ed.) *The Pituitary Gland.* pp. 405–39. (New York: Raven Press)
2. Flückiger, E., Del Pozo, E. and von Werder, K. (1982). Prolactin physiology, pharmacology and clinical findings. In *Monographs on Endocrinology.* Vol. 23. (Berlin, Heidelberg, New York: Springer)

3. Thorner, M.O., Flückiger, E. and Calne, D.B. (eds.) (1980). *Bromocriptine: A Clinical and Pharmacological Review.* (New York: Raven Press)
4. von Werder, K., Sobieszcyk, S., Schopohl, J., Scholz, A. and Horowski, R. (1987). Transdihydrolisuride (terguride) in the treatment of hyperprolactinemia. In Ratnam, S.S. and Teoh, E.S. (eds.) *Advances in Fertility and Sterility Series.* Vol. 5, pp. 169–73. (Carnforth, UK and Park Ridge, NJ, USA: Parthenon Publishing)
5. Melis, G.M., Gambacciani, M., Paoletti, A.M., Beneventi, F., Mais, V., Baroldi, P. and Fioretti, P. (1987). Dose related prolactin inhibitory effect of the new long acting dopamine receptor agonist cabergoline in normal cycling, puerperal, and hyperprolactinemic women. *J. Clin. Endocrinol. Metab.,* **65**, 541–5
6. von Werder, K. and Rjosk, H.K. (1986). Comparative effects of bromocriptine and the other dopamine agonists. In Ludwig, H. and Thomsen, K. (eds.) *Gynaecology and Obstetrics.* pp. 831–3. (Berlin, Heidelberg: Springer)
7. Mattei, A.M., Ferrari, C., Baroldi, P., Cavioni, V., Paracchi, A., Galparoli, C., Romano, D., Spellecchia, D., Gerevini, G. and Crosignani, P.G. (1988). Prolactin lowering effect of acute and once weekly repetitive oral administration of cabergoline at two dose levels in hyperprolactinemic patients. *J. Clin. Endocrinol. Metab.,* **66**, 193–8
8. von Werder, K., Landgraf, R., Müller, O.A., Rjosk, H.K. and Del Pozo, E. (1985). Treatment of hyperprolactinemia with the new dopamine agonist mesulergin (CU 32-085). In MacLeod, R.M., Thorner, M.O. and Scapagnini, U. (eds.) *Prolactin. Basic and Clinical Correlates, Fidia Research Series.* Vol. 1. (Padova: Liviana Press)
9. Varga, L., Wenner, R. and Del Pozo, E. (1973). Treatment of galactorrhea-amenorrhea syndrome with Br-ergocryptine (CB-154): restoration of ovulatory function and fertility. *Am. J. Obstet. Gynecol.,* **117**, 75–9
10. Grossman, A. and Besser, G.M. (1985). Prolactinomas. *Br. Med. J.,* **290**, 182–4
11. Chiodini, P.G., Liuzzi, A., Cozzi, R., Verde, G., Opizzi, G., Dallabonzana, D.D., Spelta, B., Sivesterini, F., Borghi, G., Luccarelli, G., Rainer, E. and Horowski, R. (1981). Size reduction of macroprolactinomas by bromocriptine or lisuride treatment. *J. Clin. Endocrinol. Metab.,* **53**, 737–43
12. Horowski, R., Dorow, R., Scholz, A., de Cecco, L. and Schneider, W.H.F. (1984). Lisuride – a new drug for treatment of hyperprolactinemic disorders. In Rolland, R. (ed.) *Advances in Fertility Control and Treatment of Sterility.* pp. 37–49. (Lancaster: MTP Press)
13. Gräf, K.J., Köhler, D., Horowski, R. and Dorow, R. (1986). Rapid regression of macroprolactinomas by the new dopamine partial agonist

terguride. *Acta Endocrinol. (Kbh.)*, **111**, 460–6
14. Landgraf, R., Rieder, G., Schmiedek, P., Clados, D., Bise, K. and von Werder, K. (1985). Hormone-active intradural spinal metastasis of a prolactinoma – a case report. *Klin. Wochenschr.*, **63**, 379–84
15. Lancranjan, I. (1986). A new approach to initiate the treatment of patients with prolactinomas. In Genazzani, A.R., Volpe, A. and Facchinetti, F. (eds.) *Gynecological Endocrinology.* pp 239–52. (Carnforth, UK and New Jersey, USA: Parthenon Publishing)
16. Montini, M., Pagani, G., Gianola, D., Pagani, M.D., Salmoiraghi, M., Ferrari, L. and Lancranjan, I. (1986). Long-lasting suppression of prolactin secretion and rapid shrinkage of prolactinomas after a long-acting, injectable form of bromocriptine. *J. Clin. Endocrinol. Metab.*, **63**, 266–8
17. Schettini, G., Lombardi, G., Merola, B., Miletto, P., Fariello, C., Cirillo, S., Fusco, R. and Lancranjan, I. (1988). Effectiveness of a single injectable dose of bromocriptine long acting in the treatment of macroprolactinomas. *J. Endocrinol. Invest.*, **11**, 47–51
18. Thorner, M.O., Martin, W.H., Rogol, A.D., Morris, J.L., Perryman, R.L., Conway, B.P., Howards, S.-S., Wolfman, M.G. and MacLeod, R.M. (1980). Rapid regression of pituitary prolactinomas during bromocriptine treatment. *J. Clin. Endocrinol. Metab.*, **51**, 438–45

5
The use of two injectable long-acting bromocriptine preparations (Parlodel® LA and Parlodel® LAR, Sandoz) in patients with prolactinoma

F. Cavagnini, C. Maraschini, M. Moro, M. De Martin, C. Invitti, A. Brunani and I. Lancranjan

---

INTRODUCTION

There is general agreement, at the present time, on the fact that dopamine receptor agonists should be employed as treatment of first choice in patients with prolactin (PRL)-secreting tumors[1,2]. This approach allows, in many patients, normalization of plasma prolactin and avoids surgical operation or, in the case of large pituitary adenomas, renders their removal easier due to the shrinkage of the tumor, that takes place in about 70% of patients treated with dopaminergic agents[3,4]. Some patients, however, are only partial responders to these drugs which, on the other hand, may be poorly tolerated by other patients[5]. In the search for more potent and better tolerated compounds, two long-acting injectable preparations of bromocriptine, Parlodel® LA[6–8] and Parlodel® LAR (Sandoz)[9,10], the latter specifically conceived for repeated administrations, have recently been developed. We compared the effectiveness and the tolerability of single injections of the two preparations on 32 patients bearing a prolactinoma. In 11 of them, treatment was continued for 2–17 months by repeated injections of Parlodel LAR.

PATIENTS AND METHODS

We investigated 32 patients, 27 women and 5 men, aged 16–66 years, bearing a PRL-secreting pituitary adenoma. 15 of them had a microadenoma (MIC), while 17 had a macroadenoma (MAC). Diagnosis was established by high resolution CT scan with enhancement and completed by visual field examination. This latter was abnormal in seven patients with MAC. One MIC and six MAC patients had previously undergone unsuccessful surgery, while 25 patients had already been treated with oral bromocriptine, which had been withdrawn at least 1 month before the study. Ten MAC and seven MIC patients were given, deeply intragluteally, a single injection of 50 mg Parlodel LA while eight MIC and seven MAC patients were injected with 50 mg Parlodel LAR. Parlodel LA and Parlodel LAR (Sandoz) contain bromocriptine microspheres employing polylactic acid in dextran solution and D,L-polylactide-co-glycolid glucose, respectively, as carrier materials. Due to the complete degradation of its vehicle in 2 months, Parlodel LAR is suitable for repeated injections. Five MIC and six MAC patients were treated with multiple injections of Parlodel LAR which was repeated in the same patient from 2 to 17 times at 4–12-week intervals. In four patients, the dose of the drug was increased up to 100 mg per injection. Plasma samples for PRL estimation were obtained prior to and, at different time intervals, after drug injection. Clinical and laboratory examination was also performed under basal conditions and during treatment. CT scan was repeated in 21/32 patients.

RESULTS

Injection of Parlodel LA and Parlodel LAR caused, in MIC and MAC patients, a prompt and steep fall of plasma PRL, whose levels lowered to about 25% of baseline already 12 h thereafter. PRL inhibition persisted for several days or weeks, re-entering in many patients into the normal limits (Figure 1). The main parameters describing the PRL pattern after the injection are summarized in Table 1. The PRL fall, expressed as percentage variation of baseline, was independent of its initial values and of the size of the tumor, while its normalization was more frequent when basal levels were only moderately increased. From

Parlodel LA and Parlodel LAR in prolactinomas

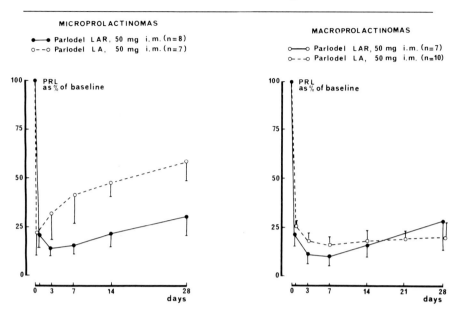

Figure 1 PRL profiles (mean ± SEM) following single injections of Parlodel LA and Parlodel LAR in patients with micro- and macroadenoma

Figure 1 and Table 1 it is readily agreed that Parlodel LAR is at least as potent as Parlodel LA in lowering plasma PRL.

By chronic administration of Parlodel LAR it was possible, in MIC and MAC patients, to induce PRL inhibition for as long as 17 months (Figures 2-4). In more detail, in two MIC (V.R. and C.A. in Figure 2) and in two MAC (R.E. and B.A. in Figure 3) patients, PRL could be steadily kept within the normal limits by monthly injections. In one patient (D.M. in Figure 4) PRL levels could be maintained steadily suppressed by an injection administered every 3 months. In another (V.M. in Figure 2) it was necessary to increase the dose of Parlodel LAR to 100 mg per injection to achieve PRL normalization. In other cases (N.R. in Figure 2, S.G. in Figure 3), there was a tendency for PRL to escape from inhibition between the monthly injections. Finally, in patients S.M. (Figure 2), F.R. and C.L. (Figure 3), PRL levels could not be suppressed to within the normal values in spite of increasing the dose of Parlodel LAR injected to 100 mg.

Shrinkage of the pituitary tumor was documented, following single or multiple administrations of Parlodel LA or Parlodel LAR, in 9/21 (three MIC and six MAC) patients in whom a control CT scan was

Table 1 Plasma PRL before and after single injection of Parlodel LA and Parlodel LAR

	Parlodel LA			Parlodel LAR	
	MIC (n = 7)	MAC (n = 10)	MIC (n = 8)		MAC (n = 7)
Basal values (ng/ml) means ± SEM	95.3 ± 18.96	573.5 ± 190.10	148.6 ± 39.00		464.7 ± 202.49
Nadir value (% of baseline)	27.3 ± 8.50	15.7 ± 4.39	14.1 ± 4.80		10.3 ± 4.09
Day of occurrence	12 h	7	3		7
Value at the 28th day (% of baseline)	58.7 ± 10.88	19.4 ± 5.15	31.0 ± 9.00		28.4 ± 14.22
Normalization	5/7 (71.4%)	3/10 (30%)	6/8 (75%)		4/7 (57.1%)

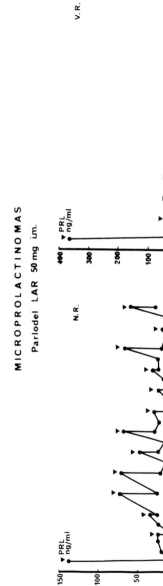
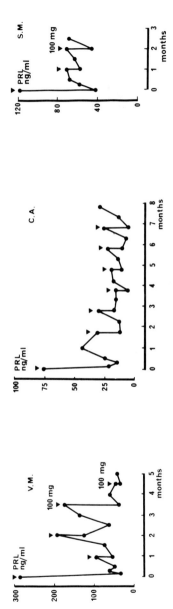

Figure 2 PRL patterns in patients with microprolactinoma treated with repeated injections of Parlodel LAR

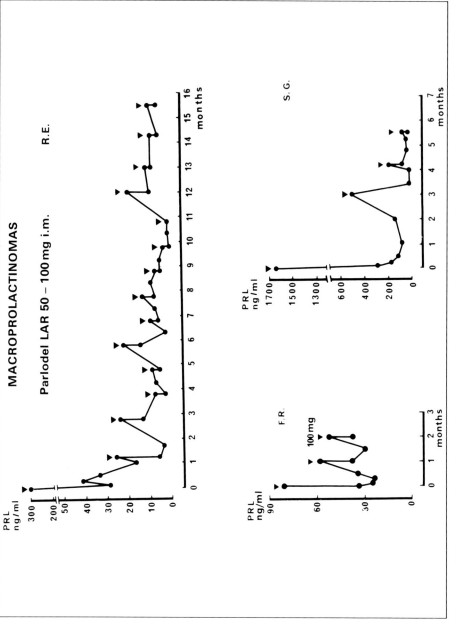

Figure 3 PRL patterns in patients with macroprolactinoma treated with repeated injections of Parlodel LAR

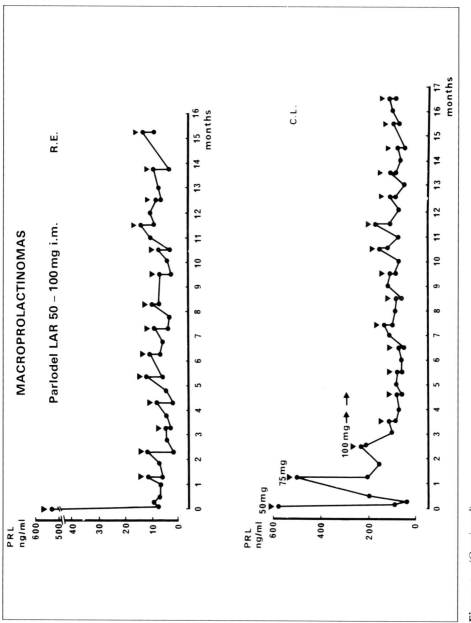

Figure 3 (Continued)

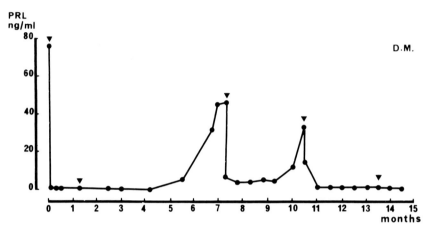

Figure 4 PRL pattern after administration of Parlodel LAR. Relevance of a proper timing of the injections

performed.

Treatment was in general well tolerated. Soreness and rash at the injection site occurred in about 10% of the patients. General side-effects such as nausea, vomiting, headache, dizziness and hypotension occurred in about 30% of the patients following the first injection of Parlodel LA or Parlodel LAR. They were limited to the injection day, were of mild or moderate degree and subsided spontaneously in a few hours. Tolerability appeared to be better in patients with MAC than in those with MIC. Finally, the incidence of side-effects decreased to about 10% with repetition of the injections.

DISCUSSION

Parlodel LA and Parlodel LAR, two long-acting injectable preparations of bromocriptine, have proved capable, in patients with prolactinoma, of producing, within a few hours from their administration, a sharp and long-lasting PRL fall[11-13]. Maximal PRL inhibition, with lowering of the hormone to approximately 15% of baseline, takes place within

1 week after the injection; 1 month thereafter, PRL levels are, on the average, still about 25% of pretreatment values. In occasional patients, plasma PRL remains steadily suppressed for 2 months or longer. As expected from the experience with oral bromocriptine[12], individual responses to the injectable formulations are unpredictable. Indeed, the PRL decrease associated with the injections, when evaluated as percentage variation from its baseline values, is independent of these latter as well as of the size of the tumor; instead, PRL normalization is more frequently achieved when its initial levels are only moderately increased. 70% of MIC patients normalized their PRL levels for variable periods of time following injection of either preparation, while in MAC patients the prevalence of normalization was slightly higher after Parlodel LAR (57%) than after Parlodel LA (30%). Comparing the PRL patterns recorded after injection of the two galenical forms, it is evident that Parlodel LAR is at least as effective as Parlodel LA in its PRL-lowering capacity[14,15].

At present, we have 11 patients who have been treated with Parlodel LAR from 2 to 17 months. In eight of them, four MIC and four MAC, it was possible, by injections given at not less than monthly intervals, to keep full normalization both of the PRL levels and of the clinical conditions, i.e. normal menses and absence of galactorrhea in women and normal sexual potency in men. One of these patients (D.M. in Figure 4) may be kept under normal laboratory and clinical conditions by an injection given every 3 months; in another (V.M. in Figure 2) 100 mg Parlodel LAR monthly is necessary to bring PRL down to within the normal values. In three patients, one MIC (S.M. in Figure 2) and two MAC (F.R. and C.L. in Figure 3), PRL is maintained well below its starting levels, but, in spite of monthly injections of 100 mg of the drug, above the normal limits.

In our patients receiving repeated injections of Parlodel LAR reduction of the tumor size could be documented by repetition of CT scan, in 2/2 MIC and in 5/6 MAC. In a collaborative study[13], the prevalence of tumor shrinkage recorded on a large series of MAC patients treated with Parlodel LAR, was of 39/54 cases (72%)[16]. In most of these patients, a reduction of the tumoral mass occurred after the first injection. Based on these observations, administration of Parlodel LAR appears to be the first measure to be taken in patients with large prolactinomas. This may allow the assessment, in a short time, of the responsiveness of PRL to bromocriptine, which requires much longer times when the drug is given orally, and a reduction of the size of the adenoma. In respect of the latter, it is worth emphasizing that shrinkage of the tumoral tissue may supervene even after several months of treatment. Tolerability of the two preparations has been, in general, definitely good; in particular, it has been slightly better in MAC than in MIC patients. Side-effects such as nausea, headache, vomiting, and dizziness and hypotension occurred in about 30% of the patients on the day of the first injection of Parlodel LAR and faded out spontaneously in a few hours. Their incidence decreased markedly with repetition of the injections[13].

On the whole, this study has demonstrated that the two long-acting injectable formulations of bromocriptine, Parlodel LA and Parlodel LAR (Sandoz) are highly effective in producing a sustained inhibition of plasma PRL levels in patients bearing a prolactinoma. Repeated injections of Parlodel LAR allow long-term treatment of these patients. Appropriate dosage and timing of the injections has to be established in individual patients. These preparations offer the physician a further tool to improve medical treatment of patients with prolactin-secreting tumors.

REFERENCES

1. Tan, S. L. and Jacobs, H. S. (1986). Management of prolactinomas – 1986. Br. J. Obstet. Gynaecol., **93**, 1025–9
2. Molitch, M. E., Elton, R. L., Blackwell, R. E., Caldwell, B., Chang, R. J., Jaffe, R., Joplin, G., Robbins, R. J., Tyson, J., Thorner, M. O. and the Bromocriptine Study Group (1985). Bromocriptine as primary therapy for prolactin-secreting macroadenomas: results of a prospective multicenter study. J. Clin. Endocrinol. Metab., **60**, 698–705
3. Demura, R., Kubo, O., Shizume, K. and Kitamura, K. (1985). Changes in computed tomographic findings in microplactinomas before and after bromocriptine. Acta Endocrinol. (Copenh.), **110**, 308–12
4. Liuzzi, A., Dallabonzana, D., Oppizzi, G., Verde, G. G., Cozzi, R., Chiodini, P. and Luccarelli, G. (1985). Low doses dopamine agonists in the long-term treatment of macroprolactinomas. N. Engl. J. Med., **313**, 656–9
5. Grossman, A., Wass, J. A. H. and Besser, M. (1987). The rapid diagnosis of sensitivity or resistance to dopamine agonists with depot-bromocriptine.

Acta Endocrinol. (Copenh.), **116**, 275–81
6. Del Pozo, E., Schluter, K., Nuesch, E., Rosenthaler, J. and Kerp, L. (1986). Pharmacokinetics of a long-acting bromocriptine preparation (Parlodel LA) and its effect on release of prolactin and growth hormone. Eur. J. Clin. Pharmacol., **29**, 615–18
7. Lancranjan, I. (1986). A new approach to initiate the treatment of patients with prolactinomas. In Genazzani, A. R., Volpe, A. and Facchinetti, F. (eds.) Gynecological Endocrinology. Proceedings of the First International Congress on Gynecological Endocrinology, pp. 239–52. (Carnforth and Park Ridge: Parthenon Publishing)
8. Montini, M., Pagani, G., Gianola, D., Pagani, M. D., Salmoiraghi, M., Ferrari, L. and Lancranjan, I. (1986). Long-lasting suppression of prolactin secretion and rapid shrinkage of prolactinomas after a long-acting injectable form of bromocriptine. J. Clin. Endocrinol. Metab., **63**, 266–8
9. Brunani, A., Maraschini, C., Invitti, C., Moro, M., Lancranjan, I. and Cavagnini, F. (1988). Chronic treatment of prolactin-secreting pituitary tumors by two long acting preparations of bromocriptine, Parlodel LA and Parlodel LAR, Sandoz. In Research on the Brain and the Female Reproductive Function. (In press)
10. Savino, L., Goffi, S., Ciccarelli, E., Ghigo, E., Bertagna, A., Gandini, G., Avataneo, T., Lancranjan, I. and Camanni, F. (1987). Long-acting bromocriptine in tumorous hyperprolactinemia treatment. J. Endocrinol. Invest., **10** (Suppl. 3), 82
11. Ciccarelli, E., Ghigo, E., Mazza, E., Andreis, M., Massara, F., Lancranjan, I. and Camanni, F. (1987). Effects of a new long-acting form of bromocriptine on tumorous hyperprolactinemia. J. Endocrinol. Invest., **10**, 179–82
12. Grossman, A., Ross, R., Wass, J. H. A. and Besser, G. M. (1986). Depot-bromocriptine treatment for prolactinomas and acromegaly. Clin. Endocrinol., **24**, 231–8
13. Lancranjan, I., Pagani, G., Cavagnini, F., Schettini, G. and Bronstein, M. (1988). Long-term treatment of prolactinomas with monthly injections of bromocriptine long-acting. In Pain and Reproduction. (Carnforth and Park Ridge: Parthenon Publishing) (In press)
14. Maraschini, C., Moro, M., Invitti, C., Brunani, A., Lancranjan, I. and Cavagnini, F. (1987). Impiego, di due preparazioni iniettabili di bromocriptina long-acting (Parlodel LA e Parlodel LAR, Sandoz) in pazienti con prolattinoma. In Prolattina '87, November, Milan, Italy
15. Pagani, G., Lancranjan, I., Nicola, G. C., Pagani, M. D., Gianola, D., Dominoni, I., Ghilardi, G., Salmoiraghi, M., Cortesi, L. and Montini, M. (1987). La bromocriptina iniettabile nel trattamento del prolattinoma:

esperienze con due nuove forme galeniche in 49 casi. In *Prolattina '87*, November, Milan, Italy
16. Lancranjan, I., Buchfelder, M., Montini. M., Schettini, G. and Cavagnini, F. (1988). Long-lasting suppression of PRL secretion and rapid and sustained shrinkage of prolactinomas after repeated injections of a long-acting injectable form of bromocriptine. *Gynecol. Endocrinol.*, **2** (Suppl. 2), 86

6
Parlodel® SRO®: an oral modified release formulation of bromocriptine with improved tolerability

J. Drewe, E. Abisch and R. Neeter

INTRODUCTION

Bromocriptine, (Parlodel[R]) (CB), is an ergot-derived dopamine agonist used in the treatment of hyperprolactinemic disorders, acromegaly and Parkinson's disease. The total daily doses employed in these indications are: 5–12.5 mg, 10–60 mg and 20–40 mg, respectively[1].

In each case, the daily dose is given in 2–4 smaller doses to decrease potential side-effects and to achieve a longer-lasting therapeutic action. These side-effects are thought to be related to the rate and extent of absorption of the drug or following formation of metabolites. In order to reduce the side-effects, an oral modified release formulation for CB is currently under development.

The present studies have been concerned with the possible influence of meals on the pharmacokinetic profiles of the oral modified release formulation (OMRF) and normal formulation (NF). In this regard, it should be noted that in clinical practice the NF of CB is recommended to be taken *during meals* in order to improve tolerability[1]. This effect may be caused by a slower absorption rate of CB in the fed state[2].

METHODS

Test articles

Study I

(1) 5 mg CB OMRF capsule (Parlodel® SRO®), Sandoz Ltd., Switzerland);

(2) 5 mg Parlodel NF capsule;

(3) Placebo capsule size 2;

(4) Placebo capsule size 1.

Study II
(1) 2.5 mg CB OMRF capsule (Parlodel® SRO®, Sandoz Ltd., Switzerland);

(2) 2.5 mg Parlodel NF capsule;

(3) Placebo capsule size 2;

(4) Placebo capsule size 1.

The release characteristics of the NF were equal with that of the commercially available standard. The OMRF was based on a swelling hydrocolloid principle and contained hydroxypropyl methylcellulose, microcrystalline cellulose and cetylpalmitate as the principal ingredients.

Study design

Studies were performed in accordance with the Declaration of Helsinki. The protocols were approved by local independent Institutional Review Boards. All subjects gave their written informed consent to the studies undertaken.

In Study I, eight, and in Study II, 18, healthy male subjects (median age 23 years, range 21–36 years; median weight 68 kg, range 56–91.3 kg) with no clinically significant pathological findings in physical examination, ECG and laboratory investigations and on no medication were studied.

Because of different capsule sizes, both formulations were taken either without or with a standardized breakfast in a four-way (study I) or a three-way (study II) cross-over, double-blind, double-dummy design.

Subjects were fasting at least 10 hours prior to drug administration. The capsules were administered at 9:00 a.m. Subjects of the fed group swallowed the capsules exactly 10 min after starting breakfast. For the first 6 hours the subjects remained in bed to avoid possible orthostatic reactions. The washout period between administrations was 7 days.

The standard breakfast consisted of: 150 ml of orange juice, two rolls,

20 g butter, 25 g marmalade, two scrambled eggs, two slices of bacon and 200 ml of whole milk. Lunch was taken 4 hours after drug administration and was also standardized for the study days. Dinner was served at 7:00 p.m. For dinner there was no special recommendation.

Fluid intake was allowed ad libitum, but was limited to fruit juice, mineral water and lemon or orange tea. The subjects had to refrain from smoking during the study.

Blood samples (volume 5 ml) were taken −3 h, −2 h, −1 h, 0 h, +20 min, 40 min, 1 h, 1.5 h, 2 h, 3 h, 4 h, 5 h, 7 h, 9.5 h, 12 h, 15 h, 17 h, 19 h, 22 h, 23 h, 24 h, 27 h, 30 h, 33 h and 36 h after drug administration. Samples were collected into heparinized tubes and separated immediately after centrifugation at 4°C and then stored at −20°C prior to analysis.

Pulse rate and blood pressure were recorded in the *supine position* prior to blood samples no. 3–13. In addition, measurements were also taken at 6 hours after administration. At this time measurements were taken immediately upon standing and after 1, 2 and 3 min standing. If any orthostatic reactions had occurred, the subjects had to remain supine until blood pressure was again in the normal range and no side-effects occurred. In this case, measurements were repeated hourly.

Analysis

PRL concentrations were analysed using a specific radioimmunoassay with a detection limit[3] of 1 ng/ml. CB plasma concentrations were analysed using a specific and sensitive radioimmunoassay with a detection limit[4] of 15 pg/ml. Blood samples no. 1–3, 17, 19, 20, 22 and 24 were only analysed for PRL.

For each regimen the maximum plasma concentration, C_{pmax}, and the time to reach maximum plasma concentration, T_{max}, were determined. The area under the plasma concentration curve AUC (0–36 h) for CB was calculated by trapezoidal rule. The values below detection limit were regarded as zero for AUC calculations. For the extrapolation of the AUC to infinity for each subject the plasma concentration curves of the fasting administration of the NF were fitted to a linear two-compartment model with first order absorption and first order elimination from the central compartment. The fitting was performed using the ELSFIT non-linear extended least-square routine[5]. For the extrapolation, the following relation was used[6]:

Table 1 Dizziness, nausea, vomiting and sickness after four different treatments with bromocriptine. Study I ($n = 8$)

	No. of subjects (severity)			
	NF fasted	NF fed	OMRF fasted	OMRF fed
Dizziness	4 (1–3) (1 drop out)	1 (2)		
Nausea	1 (2)	2 (1–2)		1 (2)
Vomiting	2 (1–3) (1 drop out)	1 (1)		
Nasal congestion	2 (2)	4 (2)	3 (2)	2 (1–2)
Sickness		3 (1–3) (1 drop out)		

Score of severity : 1 = mild; 2 = moderate; 3 = severe

Table 2 Dizziness, nausea, vomiting and sickness after three different treatments with bromocriptine. Study II ($n = 18$)

	No. of subjects (severity)		
	NF fasted	OMRF fasted	OMRF fed
Dizziness	11 (1–2)	2 (1–2)	1 (1)
Nausea	3 (2)		5 (1–3)
Vomiting	1 (2)		
Nasal congestion	10 (1–2)	3 (1)	4 (1)

Score of severity : 1 = mild; 2 = moderate; 3 = severe

$$\text{AUC}(\infty) = \text{AUC}(0-t^\star) + \int_{t}^{\infty} \star \text{Cp}(s)ds = \text{AUC}(0-t^\star) + \frac{C_p(t^\star)}{\beta}$$

where $t^\star$ denotes the last sampling point. The extrapolation was carried out under the assumption that the β-phase was not affected by the different regimens.

As a measure of the degree of retardation the half-value duration (HVD) of the plasma concentration time curves of CB was calculated, defined as follows: the total duration that values of the CB plasma concentration were above one-half of C_{pmax}. Endpoints of that time

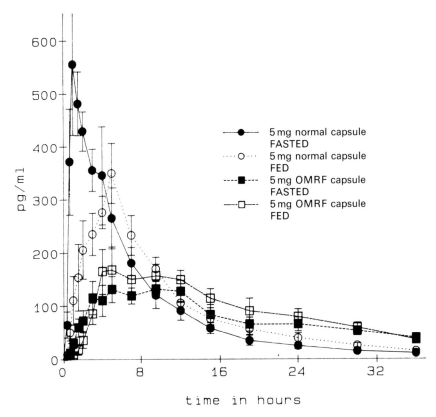

Figure 1 Mean ±SEM (pg/ml) plasma concentrations of bromocriptine ($n = 8$) after different administrations of 5 mg bromocriptine

interval were determined by linear interpolation, if necessary.

The PRL inhibition effect of CB was assessed by the area under the plasma PRL concentration curve AUC(0–36 h).

For multiple comparisons of parameters, samples were first tested for normal distribution by the Wilk–Shapiro test and for homogeneity of variances. When normal distribution of the data could not be rejected, groups were tested by two-way analysis of variance (ANOVA). In the case of significant differences, this was followed by the Newman–Keuls multicomparison test for pairwise comparisons. For not normally distributed samples, the non-parametric Friedman test was applied. All statistical tests were used as routines in RS/1, a commercially available

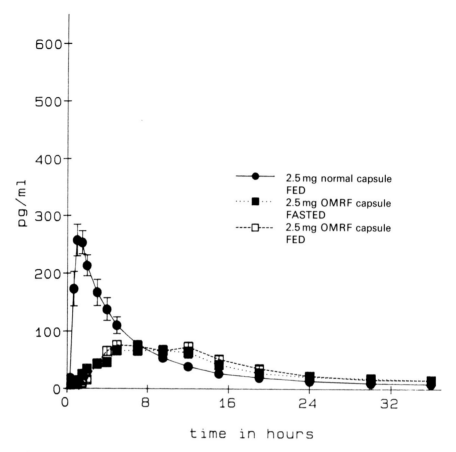

Figure 2 Mean ±SEM (pg/ml) plasma concentrations of bromocriptine ($n = 18$) after different administrations of 2.5 mg bromocriptine

software package for VAX computers[7]. The level of significance was $p = 0.05$.

RESULTS

Side-effects like dizziness, nausea, vomiting and sickness were reported with different incidence and severity after administration of the four treatments in Study I (Table 1) and Study II (Table 2).

6 hours after administration of the OMRF seven of eight volunteers

Table 3 Study I: model independent pharmacokinetic parameters

	Parameters CV (%)			
	A NF fasted	B NF fed	C OMRF fasted	D OMRF fed
AUC (inf.) (pg h ml^{-1})	3688.55 (35.0)	3603.63 (34.2)	3228.34 (40.7)	3770.82 (38.4)
Rel. biov. (%)	100	96.74 (37.2) 100	84.61 (21.3)	107.5 (43.0)
C_{pmax} (pg/ml)	691.0 (37.97)	402.38 (42.16) **a	172.13 (44.5) **a *b	206.38 (53.37) **a *b
T_{max} (h)	1.64 (67.4)	4.06 (31.1)	8.5 (43.0) **a	8.06 (50.3) **a
HVD (h)	2.79 (34.8)	5.99 (43.3)	12.93 (39.1) **a	14.76 (39.6) **a

a: significantly different from treatment A
b: significantly different from treatment B
*: $p < 0.05$; **: $p < 0.01$

could stand over a period of 3 min without experiencing any orthostatic side-effects, in comparison to four of eight with the NF in Study I. In the second study seven out of 18 subjects could stand over a period of 3 min without orthostatic symptoms after administration of the NF, 17 of 18 and 16 of 18 volunteers could do it after the administration of the OMRF under fed and fasting conditions, respectively.

The CB plasma levels for each formulation are illustrated as mean curves ($\pm$ SEM) in Figures 1 and 2. The model independent pharmacokinetic parameters are summarized in Tables 3 and 4. In both studies, no statistically significant differences in the bioavailability between the

Table 4 Study II: model independent pharmacokinetic parameters

	Parameters CV (%)		
	A NF fasted	C OMRF fasted	D OMRF fed
AUC (inf.) (pg h ml^{-1})	1661.34 (38.9)	1387.27 (58.7)	1511.12 (34.4)
Rel. biov. (%)	100	84.84 (40.8)	96.70 (37.5)
C_{pmax} (pg/ml)	288.5 (41.7)	66.0 (65.9) ★★a ★b	139.0 (22.4) ★★a ★b
T_{max} (h)	1.37 (36.5)	7.08 (43.8) ★★a	7.58 (47.5) ★★a
HVD (h)	3.32 (39.2)	11.74 (39.2) ★★a	10.84 (51.7) ★★a

a: significantly different from treatment A
b: significantly different from treatment B
★: $p < 0.05$; ★★: $p < 0.01$

OMRF and the NF were observed. However, the OMRF showed significantly smaller values of C_{pmax}, and a significantly higher degree of retardation (HVD).

The PRL plasma levels are illustrated as mean curves ($\pm$ SEM) in Figures 3 and 4. Both OMRF showed a similar extended PRL suppression over 24 hours after drug administration as the NF of the same dose given under the same meal conditions. The AUC (0–36 h) of the prolactin concentrations was not significantly different between the regimens in both studies.

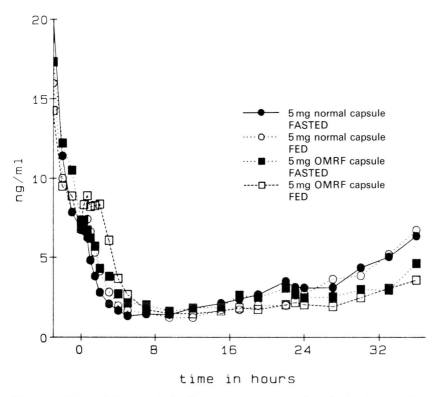

Figure 3 Mean ±SEM (pg/ml) plasma concentrations of prolactin ($n = 8$) after different administrations of 5 mg bromocriptine

DISCUSSION

Regarding the food interaction, it is remarkable that both the OMRF showed a much weaker food interaction than the NF. In Study I, the AUC was only slightly changed by food for both formulations, but the C_{pmax} of the normal capsule showed a marked food sensitivity. Under fed conditions the C_{pmax} of the NF was 48% lower than under fasting conditions, whereas for the OMRF under fed conditions C_{pmax} was even 9% higher. This might explain the clinical experience that bromocriptine NF is better tolerated when taken during a meal.

The significantly lower C_{pmax} values and the greatly retarded profile of the OMRF compared with the NF under fasting conditions will probably lead to a much lower fluctuation of plasma levels under chronic treatment.

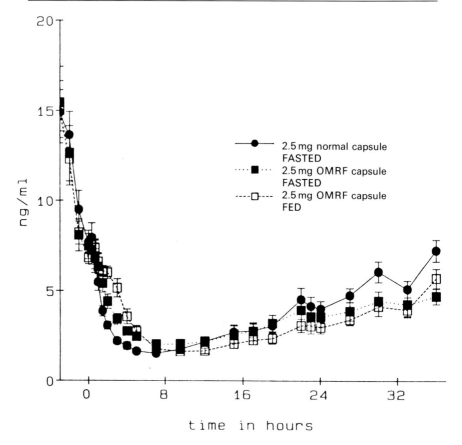

Figure 4 Mean ±SEM (pg/ml) plasma concentrations of prolactin ($n = 18$) after different administrations of 2.5 mg bromocriptine

CONCLUSION

From its improved tolerability, food insensitivity and good pharmacodynamic effect this OMRF appears to be a suitable substitute for the NF in the oral treatment with bromocriptine.

REFERENCES

1. Thorner, M.O., Flückiger, E. and Calne, D.B. (1980). *Bromocriptine. A Clinical and Pharmacological Review.* pp 55–99. (New York: Raven Press)

2. Schran, H.F., Bhuta, S.I., Schwarz, H.J. and Thorner, M.O. (1980). The pharmacokinetics of bromocriptine in man. In Goldstein, M. *et al.* (eds.) *Ergot Compounds and Brain Function: Neuroendocrine and Neuropsychiatric Aspects.* pp 125–39. (New York: Raven Press)
3. Rosenthaler, J., Munzer, H. and Voges, R. (1983). Immunoassay of bromocriptine and specificity of antibody: criteria for choice of antiserum and marker compound. In Reid, E. and Leppard, (eds.) *Drug Metabolite Isolation and Determination.* (New York: Plenum Press Corp.). Slightly modified.
4. Woodhouse, N.J.Y., Niles, N., McDonald, D. and McCorkell, S. (1985). Prolactin levels in pregnancy, comparisons of normal subjects with patients having micro- or macroadenomas after early bromocriptine withdrawal. *Horm. Res.,* **21**, 1–9
5. Sheiner, L.B. (1981). Program for the extended least squares fit to individual pharmacokinetic data. User's manual, February 1981. Division of Clinical Pharmacology, University of California, SF, USA
6. Gibaldi, M. and Perrier, D. (1982). *Pharmacokinetics.* (New York, Basle: Marcel Dekker)
7. RS/1 User's Guide (1983). BBN Research Systems. (Cambridge, Mass: Bold Beranek and Newman Inc.)

7
Parlodel® SRO® and prolactinomas: clinical and therapeutic aspects

D. Ayalon, Y. Wachsman, A. Eshel, N. Eckstein, I. Vagman and I. Lancranjan

INTRODUCTION

Prolactin-secreting pituitary adenomas are very common causes of pathological hyperprolactinemia. Medical therapy with potent dopamine receptor agonists effectively lowers raised serum prolactin levels in physiological, pharmacological and pathological hyperprolactinemia[1]. Bromocriptine has been the most widely used agent in the medical treatment of these conditions, but other drugs (all of them ergoline derivatives) proved to be almost as effective and safe, and are believed to suppress prolactin (PRL) secretion primarily by direct stimulation of pituitary dopamine receptors[2].

The majority of the dopamine agonists currently used in the treatment of hyperprolactinemia have PRL lowering effect of short duration, and their chronic use is associated frequently with side-effects such as drowsiness, sedation, headaches, postural hypotension, nausea and emesis.

The purpose of this study was therefore to evaluate the PRL lowering potency and the compliance of the hypoprolactinemic patients to the administration of a new oral modified release formulation of bromocriptine and to compare its effectiveness with two well established PRL lowering drugs – bromocriptine and lisuride.

PATIENTS AND METHODS

The study was conducted for a period of 2 months and the treatment group consisted of 21 hyperprolactinemic volunteers (19 females and 2 males). Patients who were previously treated with a PRL lowering drug underwent a washout period of at least 7 days before being included in the study. All 19 female patients had galactorrhea, and six patients amenorrhea. The chief complaints of the two male patients were impotence and loss of libido.

High resolution computed tomography (CT) scans of the pituitary area of the 21 patients revealed four macroadenomas (two males and two females) and 15 microadenomas. Two patients only had a normal CT scan.

The basal serum PRL concentrations of the treatment group ranged from 28 to 650 ng/ml (Table 1).

Design of the study

The study was carried out as an open study in two parallel groups to assess the dose–response relationships of once a day dose of Parlodel® SRO in the treatment of hyperprolactinemia. Eight patients were randomly allocated to the 2.5 mg/dose and 13 to the 5 mg/dose once daily treatment. At the end of this study (1 month's treatment with either the 2.5 mg or 5 mg dose) patients who did not achieve a normalization of serum PRL levels (<20 ng/ml) were treated for 1 more month with the 10 mg/dose Parlodel SRO once daily. On the first day of the study only, the first dose of Parlodel SRO was administered at 9.00 a.m. and nine blood samples for PRL evaluations were obtained at 8.00, 9.00, 10.00, 11.00, 12.00, 13.00, 14.00, 16.00 and 20.00 hours.

Thereafter the single dose of Parlodel SRO was administered in the evening at 20.00 hours. Blood samples for PRL evaluation were obtained also on days 2, 7 and 30 of the study at 8.00 and 9.00 hours.

All patients who were treated for an additional month of Parlodel SRO with the 10 mg/dose had blood samples taken for PRL evaluation on days 1, 7 and 30 at 8.00 and 9.00 a.m.

During the study the tolerability of the drug was assessed by measurement of vital signs (blood pressure and pulse rate) and the

Table 1 Fluctuations of serum PRL concentrations under treatment with Parlodel SRO

Group	Patient no.	Parlodel SRO daily dose (mg) (given once daily)	First month Day Time/hour														Second month (10 mg/day)					
			8	9	10	11	12	1	13	14	16	20	8	9	2	7	8	9	30	8	9	1	9	8	9	7	8	9	30	8	9

Group	Patient no.	Dose	8	9	10	11	12	1	13	14	16	20	8	9	2/9	7/8	7/9	30/8	30/9	1/8	1/9	7/8	7/9	30/8	30/9
Partial responders	1	2.5	160	131	105	155	155	122	102	71	98	155	151	71	79	92	114	87	83	110	60	75	143
	2	5.0	157	179	164	152	171	145	118	59	32	32	26	75	52	42	44	37	40	33	31	38	37
	7	2.5	86	77	70	64	67	63	50	30	26	50	48	34	47	19	24	—	—	<5	<5	<5	<5
	11	5.0	108	105	106	94	106	76	57	30	30	28	20	47	47	40	34	32	32	62	32	17	19
	19	5.0	650	700	620	670	700	1000	500	135	125	175	130	660	767	650	780	475	580	660	575	360	307
	20	5.0	103	103	101	105	104	107	91	88	81	78	91	88	97	55	68	55	68	24	64	74	64
Responders	3	5.0	32	29	29	26	24	16	11	<5	<5	<5	<5	11	12	11	17						
	4	5.0	76	64	62	60	46	45	23	12	9	<5	<5	11	12	11	17						
	5	5.0	50	56	50	49	50	45	33	27	22	39	44	8	11	18	19						
	6	2.5	84	63	80	50	60	50	43	13	10	9	8	21	24	14	21						
	8	2.5	56	62	64	48	59	58	47	38	8	<5	<5	<5	<5	<5	<5						
	9	5.0	48	54	47	43	33	32	17	13	10	<5	<5	6	6	12	13						
	10	2.5	49	45	55	49	42	29	30	21	22	11	11	6	—	—	—						
	12	5.0	53	42	41	17	13	7	<5	<5	<5	<5	<5	—	—	—	—						
	13	5.0	55	55	47	53	—	37	45	45	25	18	19	13	9	8	9						
	14	2.5	28	28	24	20	20	18	16	7	<5	<5	<5	<5	<5	<5	<5						
	15	5.0	71	78	66	71	45	—	26	—	11	15	7	10	17	6	8						
	16	2.5	66	59	64	52	72	56	57	55	57	41	39	17	22	17	22						
	17	2.5	28	24	32	40	36	34	32	27	37	23	37	12	15	14	11						
	18	5.0	105	135	100	100	100	95	77	80	64	48	46	<5	<5	<5	<5						
	21	5.0	57	52	65	42	33	22	25	18	18	22	28	9	12	21	35						

record of adverse effects.

Each patient had routine laboratory safety tests 7 days prior to admission to the study and upon completion of their participation (day 30).

RESULTS

Effect of Parlodel SRO on circulating prolactin

In nine out of 21 patients studied a normalization of PRL concentrations was obtained at 20.00 hours on the first day of treatment (<20 ng/ml) irrespective of the pretreatment, PRL concentrations and the daily dose of Parlodel SRO administered. In these patients PRL levels remained within the normal range throughout the whole period of the study (Table 1, Figure 1). Six additional patients demonstrated normal PRL levels on the 7th day of treatment. In only six patients PRL levels decreased under treatment but remained still elevated (24–780 ng/ml) at the end of the first month of treatment (partial responders). These patients (three macroadenomas and one microadenoma) had an additional month of treatment with 10 mg Parlodel SRO once a day. Under this treatment two patients (one macroadenoma and one microadenoma) normalized their PRL levels whereas two patients (two macroadenomas) had a further decrease in their PRL concentrations as compared with the PRL levels at the end of the first month of treatment. In one patient only (microadenoma) Parlodel SRO increased dose (10 mg) did not significantly lower PRL secretion (Table 1, Figure 1).

Effects on tumor mass

All patients had a 'second look' CT scan at the end of the study. Seven (35%) showed evidence of tumor regression during treatment (three macroadenomas and four microadenomas) (Figure 2).

In all the seven patients tumor shrinkage was associated with a significant fall in PRL concentrations.

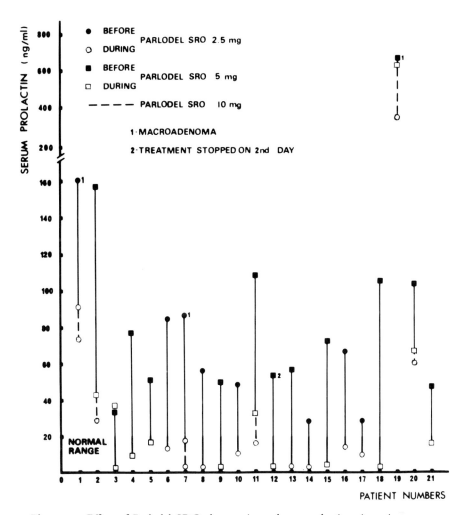

Figure 1 Effect of Parlodel SRO therapy in 21 hyperprolactinemic patients

Other PRL-lowering drugs

Lisuride

Seven patients of our series were chronically treated with lisuride, before being included in our study group. A comparative study of the PRL lowering effect of lisuride and Parlodel SRO during the first month of treatment with these two dopamine agonists has shown that

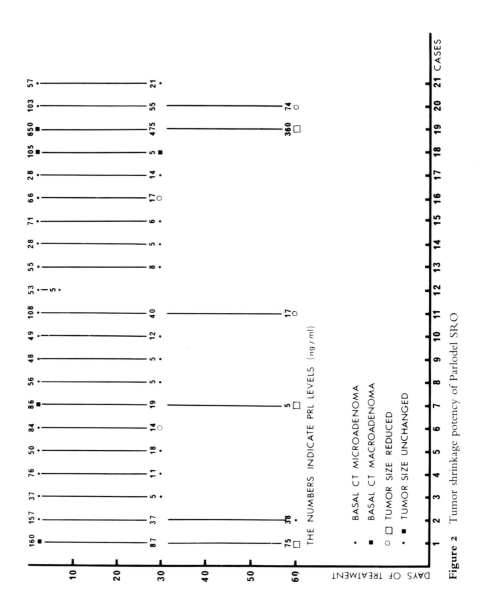

Figure 2 Tumor shrinkage potency of Parlodel SRO

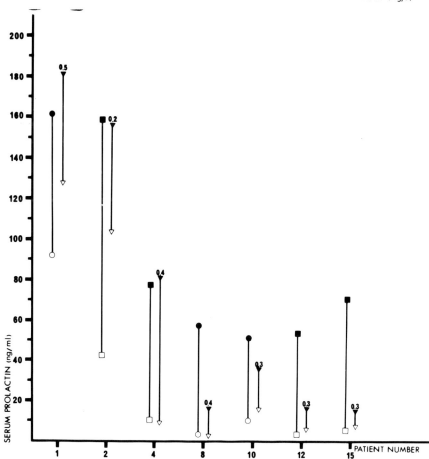

Figure 3 Effect of 1 month treatment with Parlodel SRO and lisuride on PRL levels in the same seven patients

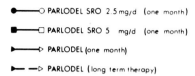

Figure 4 Circulating PRL responses to 1 month therapy with Parlodel SRO (2.5–5 mg/day), Parlodel (5–10 mg/day) and long-term therapy with Parlodel (5–15 mg/day)

Parlodel SRO (2.5–5 mg/day) is as effective as lisuride (0.2–0.5 mg/day) in the chronic treatment of hyperprolactinemic disorders (Figure 3).

Bromocriptine
The PRL lowering potency of Parlodel SRO was compared with the PRL suppressive effect of bromocriptine in six patients who were under long-term therapy with Parlodel before starting their Parlodel SRO treatment.

Our preliminary data suggest that 1 month treatment with Parlodel SRO (2.5–5 mg/day) is more effective in inhibiting PRL secretion than 1 month treatment with Parlodel (5–10 mg/day) and prolonged therapy with Parlodel (5–15 mg/day) (Figure 4).

Side-effects

Our preliminary study indicates that Parlodel SRO is well tolerated by most patients.

All patients demonstrated at the start of the treatment the classical side-effects related to the treatment with dopamine agonists, e.g. nausea, vomiting and postural hypotension. All these symptoms were usually mild and only one patient abandoned the study on the 2nd day of treatment. There were no significant changes in the laboratory safety tests performed upon completion of all the patient participations.

CONCLUSIONS

The introduction of a new and more potent ergot-related dopamine agonist, Parlodel SRO, in the treatment of hyperprolactinemic syndrome has clearly resulted in a dramatic new phase in the medical control of this endocrine entity. Parlodel SRO administered in low doses for a relatively short period of time has demonstrated its potent prolactin lowering and tumor shrinkage capacity. The inhibiting action of Parlodel SRO on PRL secretion has been shown to compare favorably with the suppressive effects of other dopamine agonists.

Parlodel SRO was well tolerated by the majority of the patients with only mild side-effects of short duration. It appears that with this new potent and longer-lasting PRL lowering agent we shall see the same clinical and biochemical effects as with the original dopamine agonist compounds, but at lower cost and with once-daily therapy.

REFERENCES

1. MacLeod, R.M. (1976). Regulation of prolactin secretion. *Front. Neuroendocrinol.*, **4**, 169–94
2. Ferrari, C. and Crosigniani, P.G. (1986). Medical treatment of hyperprolactinemic disorders. *Hum. Reprod.*, **1**, 507–14

8

Conclusions

G. M. Besser

There now appear to be a number of new potential routes of development of dopamine agonist therapy for the hyperprolactinemic syndromes. They fall into three main groups:

(1) The long-acting non-ergot derivative, CV 205-502, which may prove to provide effective once-daily therapy with a low incidence of initiating and maintenance therapy side-effects;
(2) The parenteral preparation, Parlodel LAR, which may provide suppression of circulating prolactin for a continuous period of about 4 weeks and can be given repeatedly, usually at 4-week intervals; and
(3) The modified sustained release preparation of bromocriptine itself.

This latter form (Parlodel SRO) appears to result in a slowed absorption which is delayed even more than that seen after conventional bromocriptine tablets when taken in the middle of a large bulk meal. Only if the normal formulation of bromocriptine is taken in this way are the common side-effects reduced or prevented. Perhaps the sustained release preparation will allow easier administration with less necessity for adherence to a strict 'during food' discipline, while also allowing once-daily administration.

Bromocriptine still remains the 'gold standard' for dopamine agonist medication of hyperprolactinemia, against which each new formulation or structural modification must be clinically judged. Since Ciccarelli and colleagues[1] have shown that hyperprolactinemia may be controlled in many patients by using the conventional tablets only once a day, it is clear that conclusions regarding the efficacy, incidence of side-effects and requirements for frequency of dose administration can be assessed only in double-blind cross-over studies of each new agent against conventional bromocriptine tablets given once daily. We await the outcome of such studies with eager interest since they may lead to a new and exciting phase of improved clinical care for our patients.

REFERENCE

1. Ciccarelli, E., Mazza, E., Ghigo, E., Guidoni, F., Barberis, A., Massara, F. and Camanni, F. (1987). Long-term treatment with oral single administration of bromocriptine in patients with hyperprolactinemia. *J. Endocrinol. Invest.*, **10**, 51–3

Abstracts

CV 205-502, A NOVEL OCTAHYDROBENZO[G]QUINOLINE WITH POTENT, SPECIFIC AND LONG-LASTING DOPAMINE AGONIST PROPERTIES

R.C. Gaillard, J. Brownell, K. Abeywickrama and A.F. Muller

Following the success of ergot alkaloids and their synthetic derivatives in treating hyperprolactinemia, acromegaly and parkinsonism, efforts have been concentrated on the synthesis of new derivatives and partial structures with the aim of dissecting out a specific dopaminomimetic pharmacophore. Accordingly CV 205-502 (CV), a structure which superposes the linear benzo[g]quinoline segment of apomorphine on the substituted pyrrolo[3,4-g]quinoline of the ergolines was designed. The dopaminergic properties of CV were demonstrated in vitro and in vivo in animal models. In this work, we investigated in normal volunteers 1) the effects of the compound on prolactin (PRL) and growth hormone (GH) release and 2) its site of action during a combined anterior pituitary (CAP) test using 4 hypothalamic releasing hormones (TRH 0.2 mg, GRH 0.1 mg, CRH 0.1 mg, LHRH 0.1 mg). Strong dose-dependent suppression of PRL appears following oral doses between 0.04 and 0.09 mg. A single dose of 0.06 mg given to 6 volunteers in a double-blind crossover study with placebo markedly suppressed PRL for more than 24 h, and the PRL peaks of the normal sleep profile were abolished. Three groups of 5 men were treated once daily with CV (0.04, 0.06, 0.08 mg/day) and on day 6 the CAP test was performed. One month later the test was repeated for control values. TSH, ACTH, cortisol, PRL, GH, LH, FSH and testosterone were measured. All subjects responded normally with marked increases in all hormones, both following CV treatment and after 1 month washout, with the exception of PRL response which was largely attenuated during treatment with all doses of CV (inhibition 76, 93 and 94%). These results confirm the strong dopamine agonist properties of CV and implicate the pituitary as its major site of action. These data also suggest that lactotropic cells are the only adenohypophyseal cells whose secretory activity is altered by a direct action of this dopaminergic compound.

CV 205-502, A NEW LONG-ACTING DOPAMINE AGONIST FOR THE TREATMENT OF HYPERPROLACTINEMIA: CLINICAL EXPERIENCE AND HORMONAL FINDINGS IN A 3-MONTH STUDY IN HYPERPROLACTINEMIC WOMEN

P.F.M. van der Heijden, R. Rolland, R.E. Lappøhn, R.S. Corbeij, W.B.K.M.V. de Goeij and J. Brownell

Forty-one hyperprolactinemic women have been treated for three months with the new dopamine agonist benzo[g]quinoline (CV 205-502) (CV) in a dose titration and safety study. Weeks 1–4 were conducted double blind with 20 of the women randomly assigned to once daily placebo treatment and 21 women to treatment with CV at a dose of 0.05 mg daily. From week 5 on the placebo starters also received 0.05 mg CV daily with food at bedtime. At 4-week intervals the daily CV dose could be increased by 0.025 mg to a maximum of 0.10 mg daily if serum prolactin had not normalized. Clinical evaluation and prolactin determinations were performed every 2 weeks, full laboratory and ECG safety tests every 4 weeks. At the end of treatment the following CV dose distribution/prolactin normalization had been reached: n = 20, 0.05 mg; n = 10, 0.075 mg and n = 3, 0.10 mg. The remaining 8 patients required 0.125 or 0.150 mg daily to achieve normal prolactin and they were treated beyond the period of 3 months. Of 38 women treated previously with Parlodel® 28 responded clinically as well to CV as to their previous treatment, while 10 responded better to CV. Adverse reactions were reported most often at the beginning of treatment in both groups and were slight to moderate in severity and transient in nature. In no case was discontinuation of treatment necessary. No drug-attributable abnormalities in any measure of physical, ECG or laboratory blood and urine tests were seen during the 3-month study.

ORAL AND PARENTERAL DOPAMINE AGONISTS: COMPARATIVE EFFECTS

K. von Werder, J. Schopohl and G. Mehltretter

Ergot alkaloids and their derivatives interact with adrenoreceptors, 5-HT- and DA-receptors. The prolactin (PRL) inhibitory effect of ergot derivatives is mediated by the DA_2 receptors, which are not linked to the adenyl cyclase system. The ergot compounds can be divided into 3 groups according to their structure. Bromocriptine belongs to the lysergic acid amines, pergolide and methergoline to the clavine family, whereas lisuride and terguride belong to the 8α-aminoergolines.

Most of our knowledge in treating hyperprolactinemia has derived from the experience with bromocriptine. Though oral bromocriptine is effective in more than 90% of patients with hyperprolactinemia, there are still patients, who may not tolerate the drug because of side-effects, mainly hypotension and gastrointestinal disturbances, which are intrinsic of DA receptor stimulation. Pergolide, which is 100 times more potent than bromocriptine compared on a weight basis, has similar side-effects in comparable PRL lowering dosages. Lisuride, 13 times more potent than bromocriptine, also has comparable side-effects. The transdihydroderivative of the latter compound, terguride, seems to be less active than lisuride, but has been shown to have fewer side-effects in a number of patients. However, there is pronounced individual variation. Whereas one patient may tolerate one ergot and not the others, another patient may be intolerant just of this particular compound.

All ergots with dopamine agonistic activity have been taken orally, which may explain the occasionally pronounced side-effects. Parenteral administration of dopamine agonists may therefore represent an advantage. Thus, the now available long-acting bromocriptine, which can be injected repeatedly (Parlodel® LAR) has been shown to lower

PRL levels over a period of up to 4 weeks, but is also well tolerated. Parlodel LAR is effective in micro- and macroprolactinoma patients and a double-blind study comparing oral and i.m. bromocriptine is now undertaken.

THE USE OF TWO INJECTABLE LONG-ACTING BROMOCRIPTINE PREPARATIONS (PARLODEL® LA AND PARLODEL® LAR, SANDOZ) IN PATIENTS WITH PROLACTINOMA

F. Cavagnini, C. Maraschini, M. Moro, M. de Martin, C. Invitti, A. Brunani and I. Lancranjan

The effectiveness and tolerability of two injectable long-acting preparations of bromocriptine, Parlodel® LA and Parlodel® LAR (Sandoz), the latter developed for repeatable administrations, were evaluated in 28 patients (pts.), 23 women and 5 men, bearing a prolactinoma. The pituitary tumor was demonstrated by high resolution CT scan with enhancement.

Study design

Seven pts. with micro-(MIC) and 10 with macroprolactinoma (MAC) received a single i.m. injection of Parlodel LAR 50 mg. Five pts. with MIC and 6 with MAC were injected with Parlodel LAR 50 mg; in 10 of these pts., treatment was continued for 5–13 months with injections repeated at 4–8 week intervals. In two pts., the dose of Parlodel LAR was increased, during treatment, to 100 mg/injection. CT scan was repeated in 23 pts. while on treatment.

Results

Single injections of Parlodel LA and LAR: A prompt and marked prolactin (PRL) fall occurred in the two groups of pts. following administration of either preparation (nadir $27.3 \pm 8.5\%$ of baseline at 12 h in MIC and $15.6 \pm 4.39\%$ on day 7 in MAC with Parlodel LA; $12.0 \pm 3.9\%$ in MIC and $6.6 \pm 2.19\%$ in MAC on day 7 with Parlodel LAR). Plasma PRL remained inhibited over the one month observation period following the injection ($58.7 \pm 10.88\%$ of baseline in MIC and

$19.4 \pm 5.15\%$ in MAC with Parlodel LA and $25.7 \pm 11.28\%$ in MIC and $21.1 \pm 13.79\%$ in MAC with Parlodel LAR, on the 28th day). PRL suppression appeared to be more sustained in MAC than in MIC pts., chiefly after injection of Parlodel LA. Especially in MIC pts., Parlodel LAR caused a greater PRL suppression than did Parlodel LA.

Multiple injections of Parlodel LAR: In the 10 pts. studied it was possible, by repeated injections of 50–100 mg Parlodel LAR given at 4–8 week intervals, to keep plasma PRL inhibited over the whole period of treatment (5–13 months). Plasma PRL normalized in 4/5 MIC and 3/5 MAC pts. Tumor shrinkage occurred in 3/15 pts. (1 MIC, 2 MAC) after single injection of Parlodel LA and in 6/8 pts. (2 MIC, 4 MAC) while on treatment with Parlodel LAR. Side-effects such as headache, dizziness, nausea and, occasionally, vomiting lasting a few minutes or hours occurred in about 30% of the pts. on the injection day only. They became less frequent with the subsequent injections.

Conclusions

The two injectable preparations of bromocriptine, Parlodel LA and Parlodel LAR, allow a sustained suppression of plasma PRL in pts. with prolactinoma. By repeated injections of Parlodel LAR it is possible, in the majority of these pts. to keep PRL levels within the normal range.

PARLODEL® SRO®: AN ORAL MODIFIED RELEASE FORMULATION OF BROMOCRIPTINE WITH IMPROVED TOLERABILITY

J. Drewe, E. Abisch and R. Neeter

Bromocriptine (CB) is an ergot derived dopamine agonist used in the treatment of hyperprolactinemic disorders, in acromegaly and Parkinson's disease. To reduce the incidence and severity of its dose-dependent side-effects (e.g. nausea, vomiting, dizziness, nasal congestions and orthostatic reactions) which may occur especially in the first phase of treatment, an oral modified release formulation (OMRF) for bromocriptine (Parlodel® SRO®) is currently under development.

Methods

In two human studies in 8 and 18 healthy male volunteers a 5 mg and a 2.5 mg OMRF have been studied, respectively. In the first study the 5 mg OMRF and a 5 mg normal (instantaneous release) capsule (NF) were given as a single dose under fasting conditions and after a high fat meal. In the second study the 2.5 mg OMRF was likewise given under fed and fasting conditions, whereas the 2.5 mg NF was given only under fasting conditions. In both studies blood samples for bromocriptine and prolactin determination were drawn and blood pressure and pulse rate were measured before and up to 36 and 7 hours after administration, respectively.

Results

In the first study the incidence and intensity of side-effects were significantly smaller for the OMRF (2 times, moderate) than for the NF (10 times, moderate to severe). The relative bioavailability of the OMRF was $107.5 \pm 43.0\%$ (CV) and $84.6 \pm 21.3\%$ (CV) under fed and fasting conditions, respectively. In contrast to the virtually unchanged pharmacokinetic profile of the OMRF, the profile of the NF (rate of absorption) was markedly affected by food. Both formulations showed an extended suppression of prolactin over 36 hours in all subjects under either meal conditions. In the second study the relative bioavailability of the 2.5 mg OMRF was $96.7 \pm 37.5\%$ (CV) and $84.8 \pm 40.8\%$ (CV) under fed and fasting conditions, respectively. The insensitivity to food could be confirmed for this OMRF. Both formulations were well tolerated. For both formulations prolactin secretion was suppressed over 24 hours.

Conclusion

From its improved tolerability, food insensitivity and good pharmacodynamic effect (prolactin suppression) this OMRF appears to be suitable to substitute the NF in the oral treatment.

PARLODEL SRO AND PROLACTINOMAS: CLINICAL AND THERAPEUTIC ASPECTS

D. Ayalon, Y. Wachsman, A. Eshel, N. Eckstein, I. Vagman and I. Lancranjan

Twenty one hyperprolactinemic patients (19 females and 2 males) were treated for one month with Parlodel® SRO® at a daily dose of either 2.5 mg (8 patients) or 5 mg (13 patients). Before treatment a CT scan study revealed microadenomas in 18 patients and macroadenomas in 3 patients. All 19 female patients had galactorrhea associated in 6 patients with amenorrhea. Impotence was the chief complaint of the 2 male patients. Following the first month of treatment a normalization of prolactin concentration (< 20 ng/ml) was observed in 15 patients (six treated with 2.5 mg/day and 9 with 5 mg/day). Out of the 6 remaining non-responder patients 3 had macroadenomas. Following an additional month of treatment with Parlodel SRO (10 mg/day) 4 patients (2 macroadenomas and 2 microadenomas) normalized their prolactin levels. Radiological evidence of hypodense areas and tumor shrinkage was found in 7 patients. The treatment was in general well tolerated and side-effects (nausea and fatigue) were mild and usually limited to the first 10 days of treatment. Only one patient discontinued treatment after 2 days for complaints of severe dizziness.

Index

absorption rate 59
acne 32
acromegaly
   –cold-sensitive digital
      vasospasm 38
   –dopamine agonists 11
   –dose used 59
   –ergot alkaloids 13
   –Parlodel® 59
   –side-effects 38
   –treatment 11
action of drugs
   –duration 16–18
   –specific 11
   –sustained 11, 16
adenohypophyseal cells 20, 23
adenomas
   –macro- 38, 48, 72
   –micro- 8, 72
   –pituitary 47, 71
administration
   –during meals 59
   –normal formulation 59
   –oral 37
   –oral modified release
      formulation 59
   –parenteral 38, 40
adrenocorticotrophic hormone 20, 23
adrenoceptors 35
alkaloids 13, 35
   –structure 36
alternative drugs 11
   –side-effects 11

–toxicity 11
amenorrhea 32, 72
   –reversal 32
8α-aminoergoline 35
anovulation 32
anterior pituitary
   hormones 18, 37
apomorphine 13

benzo[g]quinoline 13, 27
bioavailability 11
blood chemistry 28
blood pressure
   –standing 28, 33, 61, 72
   –supine 23, 28, 31, 61, 72
bromocriptine
   –absorption rate 59
   –equivalent dosages 37
   –food interactions 67
   –hyperprolactinemia 27
   –intolerance 28
   –lactation inhibition 33
   –long-acting injectables 40
   –long-term therapy 39
   –meals 59
   –oral administration 37, 59
   –Parlodel® 27, 59, 71
   –plasma concentration 63, 64
   –prolactin 11
   –prolactinoma 37
   –retardation 63
   –side-effects 27, 37
   –structure 35

—tolerance 37
—tumor shrinkage 41

cabergoline 35, 37
cerebellar metastases 38, 41
cetylpalmitate 60
clavine 35
cold-sensitive digital
   vasospasm 38
combined anterior pituitary
   function test 20
computed tomography (CT)
   48, 72
corticotropin releasing
   factor 20
cortisol plasma levels 18, 20, 23
cost 11
CU 32-085 (mesulergine) 38, 39
CV 205-502
   —acceptability 34
   —action 16, 18
   —adenohypophyseal cells 20, 23
   —adrenocorticotrophic hormone
      20
   —adverse reactions 23
   —anterior pituitary hormones 18
   —comparison with bromocriptine
      32, 33
   —cortisol 18, 20
   —discontinuation 32
   —dose 14–16, 23, 29, 34
   —duration 16–18
   —efficacy 34
   —endocrine profile 18–23
   —follicle stimulating
      hormone 18, 20, 22
   —gonadotropin 20
   —healthy subjects 13–26
   —hyperprolactinemia 27–33
   —hyperthalamic releasing
      hormone 20

   —luteinizing hormone 18, 20, 22
   —LHRH 22
   —normalized prolactin levels 29
   —pituitary 23
   —plasma growth hormone
      16–18, 20
   —plasma prolactin 15, 20
   —prolactin suppression 27
   —properties 23
   —receptor binding 13
   —safety 27–33
   —side-effects 16, 25, 32
   —single dose 27
   —sleep surges 17
   —structure 13, 14
   —testosterone 20, 22
   —thyroid 20
   —thyroid stimulating hormone
      18, 20
   —tolerance 16, 23–25, 27–33
   —TRH 24
cytotoxic therapy 41

Declaration of Helsinki 60
dihydroergocriptine 37
dizziness 32, 62–65
dopamine
   —coexistence with gonadotropin
      releasing hormone 20
   —inhibition of somatostatin
      neurons 18
   —presence in tuberoinfundibular
      system 20
   —receptors 18
   —stimulation of somatotropic
      dopamine receptors 18
dopamine agonists
   —acromegaly 11
   —action 13
   —adverse reactions 13
   —8α-aminoergolines 35

Index

–carbergoline 35
–clavine 55
–duration of effect 71
–equivalent dosages 37
–growth hormone 17
–hyperprolactinemia 11
–lactotrophs 33
–lergotrile 35
–lisuride 35
–lysergic acid amine 35
–mesulergine 35
–metergoline 35
–novel 13
–Parkinsonism 11
–pergolide 35
–prolactin 11
–side-effects 37, 71
–structure 13, 14, 36
–terguride 35, 38
–tolerance 37, 38
–variation 35
–CV 205-502 14, 37
–equivalent dosages 37
–normoprolactinemia 33
–Parlodel LA 48
–Parlodel LAR 48
–Parlodel SRO 72
–prolactin inhibition 14
–single dose 14, 27
–tolerance 14
–variation 55
double-blind trials
–CV 205-502 28
–Parlodel SRO 60
drowsiness 71
duration of action
–CV 205-502 16–18
–dopamine agonists 71
–Parlodel SRO 79

efficacy

–Parlodel LA 44, 47–56
–Parlodel LAR 44, 47–56
equivalent dosages 37
ergolines 13, 27
ergot compounds
–adverse reactions 13
–alkaloids 13, 35
–alternative drugs 11
–chronic therapy 13
–CV 205-502 34
–intolerance 23
–resistance 23
–side-effects 11
–structure 35, 36
–toxicity 11

fainting 25
fasting 60
follicle stimulating hormone 18
–LHRH 22
–plasma levels 18, 20
food interaction 67
–side-effects 81

galactorrhea 29, 32, 55, 72
gastrointestinal disorders 25, 37
gonadotropins 11
growth hormone 16
–CV 205-502 16, 18
–dopamine 20
–plasma levels 20
–releasing factor 20
–tuberoinfundibular system 20

headache 16, 23, 25, 32, 37, 71
hematology 28
hydroxypropyl methylcellulose 60
hyperprolactinemia
–CV 205-502 23, 27–34
–dose used 59
–ergot alkaloids 13, 35

–Parlodel® 59
–prolactin levels 39
–treatment 27, 35, 39
hypotension 37, 41
–postural 61, 71, 79
hypothalamus
  –anterior pituitary cells 20
  –pituitary–hypothalamic function 11
  –release hormones 20

impaired sexual function 23
impotence 72
individual responses 55
infertility 29
injectable dopamine agonists 40, 47
intolerance
  –bromocriptine 28
  –dopamine agonists 27
  –oral administration 44
intramuscular injection
  –Parlodel LA 40
  –Parlodel LAR 40

lactation
  –bromocriptine 33
  –inhibition 33
lactotroph cells 20
  –dopamine agonists 33
lergotrile 35
libido, loss of 72
lisuride 35–38, 40, 71–79
  –comparison with bromocriptine 38
  –comparison with Parlodel SRO 71, 75, 77
long-acting injectables 40–45, 47-56
long-term therapy 39
luteinizing hormone 18
  –releasing hormone 20
    FSH 22
    testosterone 22
lysergic acid amine 38

macroadenomas 38, 48, 72
macroprolactinomas 40
microadenomas 48, 72
microspheres 48
meals 59
mesulergine (CU 32-085) 35, 37
  –long-term therapy 39
  –side-effects 38
  –withdrawal 38
metastases 38, 41
metergoline 35
monthly injections 49

nasal stuffiness 37, 62–65
nausea 16, 23, 25, 32, 62–65, 71, 79
normoprolactinemia
  –CV 205-502 33
novel dopamine agonists 13

oligomenorrhea 29
oral administration 37
oral modified release formulation 59–68
orthostatic blood pressure 23, 61

parenteral administration 40, 44
Parkinsonism
  –dopamine agonists 11
  –dose used 59
  –ergot alkaloids 13
  –Parlodel® 59
  –treatment 11
Parlodel® 27
Parlodel LA 40–44
Parlodel LAR 40–44
Parlodel SRO
  –administration method 60
  –comparison with

Index

bromocriptine 71, 78, 79
- comparison with lisuride 71, 75, 77
- compliance 71–79
- dose–response relationship 72
- duration of action 79
- effect on tumor mass 74, 76
- food interaction 81
- prolactin serum levels 73, 74
- prolactinomas 71–79
- side-effects 59–68
- tolerance 59, 72, 79

pergolide 35, 37

pituitary
- adenoma 47, 71
  adrenal axis 20, 23
- challenge test 28
- CV 205-502 23
- dopamine receptors 71
  gonadal axis 20
  hypothalamic function 11
  thyroid axis 20
- TRH 28

potency 37

pregnancy 32

prolactin
- adenomas secreting prolactin 71
- bromocriptine 11
- dopamine 11
- inhibition
  CV 205-502 20, 27–33
  dose 14–16, 37
  duration 16–18, 40, 48, 56
  Parlodel LA 40–44, 48–56
  Parlodel LAR 40–44, 48–56
- measurement 28
- normalization 29–31, 40, 47, 55, 72, 74
- plasma levels 15, 20, 48
- serum levels 29, 31, 73, 74
- sleep 16

- sleep surges 17
- spontaneous release 33
- TRH 20, 21, 30, 33
- variation in response 55

prolactinoma 37, 38
- macro- 40
- malignant 38, 41
- micro- 40
- treatment 47

pulse rate 23, 28, 33, 61, 72

pyrrolo [3, 4-g] quinoline 13

radioimmunoassay 28, 61

safety
- CV 205-502 27–33

sedation 71

serotonin receptors 35

serum levels of prolactin
- dose of CV 205-502 30
- normalized 29, 31
- Parlodel SRO 73
- TRH challenge test 30

sexual potency 55

shrinkage of tumors 41, 47, 49, 55, 74, 76

side-effects
- acne 32
- blood pressure 23, 33, 37
- bromocriptine 37
- causes 59
- cold-sensitive digital vasospasm 30
- dizziness 32, 54, 62, 65
- dopamine agonists 27
- drowsiness 71
- duration 56
- fainting 25
- gastrointestinal disorders 25, 37
- headache 16, 23, 25, 32, 37, 54, 71

—hypotension 37, 41, 54, 71, 79
—lergotrile 35
—meals 59–67, 81
—nasal stuffiness 37, 62–65
—nausea 16, 23, 25, 32, 54, 62–65, 71, 79
—orthostatic reactions 61–66
—Parlodel LA 40, 44
—Parlodel LAR 40, 44
—Parlodel SRO 59–65
—potency 37
—pulse rate 23, 33
—rash 54
—sedation 71
—soreness 54
—tiredness 32
—vomiting 16, 25, 54, 62–65, 79
—weakness 25
—withdrawal 38
single dose CV 205-502 14, 27
sleep 16
sleep surges 17
somatostatin 41
somatostatin neurons 18
somatotropic dopamine receptors 38
spinal metastases 38
sterility, hyperprolactinemic 38
surgery, avoidance of 47
sustained inhibition of plasma prolactin 56
swelling hydrocolloids 60

terguride 35, 37, 38
testosterone 20
—LHRH 22
thyroid stimulating hormone 18
—CV 205-502 19, 23
—inhibition 19, 23
—measurement 28
—releasing hormone 20

—response 29
—TRH 24
tiredness 32
tolerance
—bromocriptine 27, 28–33, 37, 38
—dopamine agonists 27, 37, 38
—improvement of 37
—oral modified release formulation 68
—Parlodel® 27
—Parlodel LA 44, 47–56
—Parlodel LAR 44, 47–56
—Parlodel SRO 68, 72, 79
—terguride 38
tomography, high resolution computed 72
toxicity 11
TRH 20, 21
—challenge test 30
—pituitary challenge test 28
—plasma prolactin 21
—response 29
—serum prolactin 30, 33
—TSH 24
tuberoinfundibular system 20
tumor
—malignant 38, 41
—shrinkage 41, 49, 55, 74, 76
—see adenoma

urine analysis 28

variation in response 55
vasospasm, cold-sensitive 38
vomiting 23, 25, 62–65, 79

weakness 25
weight 28
withdrawal due to side-effects 38